Learning Medicine

Eighteenth Edition: How to Become and Remain a Good Doctor

Learning Medicine is a must-read for anyone thinking of a career in medicine, or who is already in the training process and wants to understand and explore the various options and alternatives along the way. Whatever your background, whether you are school-leaver or mature student, if you are interested in finding out more about becoming and being a good doctor, this is the book for you.

In continuous publication since 1983, and now in its eighteenth edition, *Learning Medicine* provides the most current, honest and informative source of essential knowledge combined with pragmatic guidance.

Learning Medicine describes medical school courses, explains Foundation years and outlines the wide range of specialty choices allowing tomorrow's doctors to decide about their future careers; but it also goes further to consider the privilege and responsibility of being a doctor, providing food for thought and reflection throughout a long and rewarding career.

From reviews of previous editions:

"This little volume contains everything that is required by the aspirant in medical training and also answers questions that probably would not be thought about. Particularly valuable are the details of specialisation and the requirements for this. This little volume is a must for all students (and their parents!)."

Scottish Medical Journal

"Wise, well observed and accurate (not to mention funny!). Rather than just telling you how to get into medical school – this book asks you the much more important question: "Will you enjoy it?""

Foundation Year 1 Doctor

"…provides a very objective and balanced up-to-date analysis of both medical school and medicine as a career. It not only gives the potential medical student invaluable information about what medical school is really like from day to day, and the careers it could lead to, but also help with decisions such as "is medicine for me?" and "how do I get in?"."

UCL Medical Student Clinical Year 2

"To read this is to be warned, informed and educated – a very useful piece of ground-work before even applying to medical school."

GP and GP Trainer

Learning Medicine

How to Become and Remain a Good Doctor

Eighteenth Edition

Peter Richards MA MD PhD FRCP FMEDSCI
Past President, Hughes Hall, Cambridge

Simon Stockill BSc (Hons) MB BS DCH MRCGP
General Practitioner, Leeds

Rosalind Foster BA
Barrister at Law, 2 Temple Gardens, London

Elizabeth Ingall BA MB BChir
Foundation Year 1 Doctor

*With cartoons by the late Larry
and a foreword by Sir Roger Bannister*

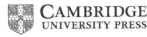

CAMBRIDGE
UNIVERSITY PRESS

University Printing House, Cambridge CB2 8BS, United Kingdom

Published in the United States of America by Cambridge University Press, New York

Cambridge University Press is part of the University of Cambridge.

It furthers the University's mission by disseminating knowledge in the pursuit of education, learning and research at the highest international levels of excellence.

www.cambridge.org
Information on this title: www.cambridge.org/9780521709675

First published 1983 by BMJ Publishing Group
Second edition 1985, 2012; third edition 1986; fourth edition 1987; fifth edition 1988;
sixth edition 1989; seventh edition 1990; eighth edition 1991; ninth edition 1992;
tenth edition 1993; eleventh edition 1994; twelfth edition 1995; thirteenth edition 1996;
fourteenth edition 1997; fifteenth edition 2000; sixteenth edition 2003;
seventeenth edition 2006

Eighteenth edition published 2008 by Cambridge University Press
First published 2011
4th printing 2012
Reprinted 2013

A catalogue record for this publication is available from the British Library

ISBN 978-0-521-70967-5 Paperback

To spirited students, dedicated doctors, and courageous and forbearing patients – all of whom have helped us to learn medicine.

With our special thanks to all those (students of several medical schools, a patient, and a BBC TV producer) who have each contributed their piece to this book – Tom Alport, Chloe-Maryse Baxter, Michael Brady, Sarah Cooper, Sarah Edwards, Adam Harrison, Farhad Islam, Liz James, Grace Robinson, Susan Spindler, Brenda Strachan, Helena Watson, Lynne Harris, David Carter, Sarah Vepers – and particularly to the late Larry, who most generously breathed life into a "worthy cause", and to his widow, who has not only kindly given us permission to continue to use the original cartoons but also to use some not previously included. We also gratefully acknowledge the assistance of Dr Aneil Malhotra in the updating of this 18th edition.

Contents

Foreword

By Sir Roger Bannister, CBE DM FRCP

The authors between them have more or less seen it all. This book gives a vivid, and fair picture of medical student life and what is involved in becoming a doctor. There is fun and esprit de corps; hard work and even drudgery.

It is also about what it means to be a doctor: the privileges and responsibilities; and about career options and pathways.

If, after carefully considering the issues raised here, you choose medicine and if you are successful in getting a place at medical school, you will be on the threshold of one profession, above all others, acknowledged all over the world to have brought the greatest advances and the greatest benefits to mankind. Medicine has fascination; it has diversity.

For 40 years I have been a neurologist and have never for one day lost the feeling of exhilaration of solving a new clinical problem. Medicine has happily been the core of my life. Study and reflect on this book and medicine might, or might not, become the core of yours too.

If you choose to represent the various parts in life by holes upon a table, of different shapes – some circular, some square, some oblong – and the persons acting these parts by bits of wood of similar shapes, we shall generally find that the triangular person has got into the square hole, the oblong in the triangular, and a square person has squeezed himself into the round hole. The officer and the office, the doer and the thing done, seldom fit so exactly that we can say they were almost made for each other.

SYDNEY SMITH 1804

If we offend, it is with good will,
That you should think we come not to offend,
but with good will

A Midsummer Night's Dream
SHAKESPEARE

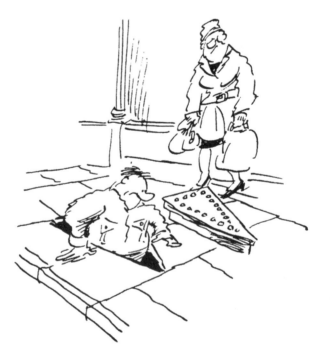

Preface

For 25 years this book, regularly updated, has assisted many people like yourself, to make your own informed decision as to whether, or not, medicine is the right career for you.

However, this book has a much wider purpose. It charts the various medical school courses, explains the Foundation years, and outlines the wide range of medical specialty choices.

Further, through its consideration of the legal consequences of the privilege and responsibility of being a doctor, it gives food for thought and reflection throughout your career in convenient bedside reading!

It also provides a readable source of information for patients and the public, about what it takes to become and remain a good doctor.

With the ever-increasing radical changes to medical education and medical practice, Medicine continues to go through difficult times, but patients will always need good doctors.

Medicine is not just another job: it is a way of life. Most doctors are highly regarded by their patients. Medicine is a tremendous career for the right people.

You will need to consider all the personal and professional implications of a life dedicated to putting patients and patient safety first.

We celebrate our 25th anniversary by sub-titling this book "How to become and remain a good doctor", to reflect its now much wider scope.

The authors

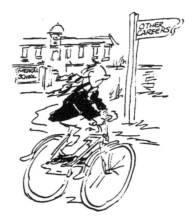

Why medicine and why not?

So you are thinking of becoming a doctor? But are you quite sure that you know what you are letting yourself in for? You need to look at yourself and look at the job. Working conditions and the training itself are improving, but medicine remains a harder taskmaster than most occupations. Doctors have also never been under greater pressure nor been more concerned for the future of the National Health Service (NHS).

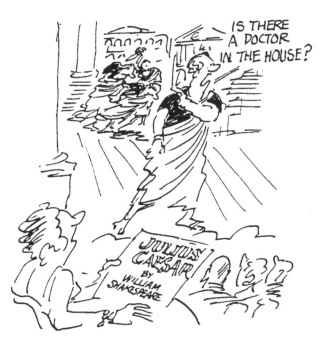

Before starting medicine you really do need to think about what lies ahead. The trouble is that it is almost impossible to understand fully what the profession demands, particularly during the early years of postgraduate training, without actually doing it. Becoming a doctor is a calculated risk because it may be at least 5 or 6 years' hard grind before you begin to discover for sure whether or not you suit medicine and it suits you. And you may change; you might like it now, at your present age and in your current frame of mind, but in 6 years' time other pressures and priorities may have crowded into your life.

Medicine is both a university education and a professional training. The first 5 or 6 years lead to a medical degree, which becomes a licence to practise. That is followed by at least as long again in practical postgraduate training. The medical degree course at university is too long, too expensive (about £200,000 in university and NHS costs, quite apart from personal costs), and too scarce an opportunity to be used merely as an education for life.

It might seem odd not to start considering "medicine or not?" by weighing up academic credentials and chances of admission to medical school. Not so; of course academic and other attributes are necessary, but there is a real danger that bright but unsuited people, encouraged by ambitious schools, parents or their own personalities, will go for a high-profile course like medicine without having considered carefully first just where it is leading. A few years later they find themselves on a conveyor belt from which it becomes increasingly difficult to step. Could inappropriate selection of students (most of whom are so gifted that they almost select themselves) account for disillusioned doctors? Think hard about the career first and consider the entry requirements afterwards.

Getting into medical school and even obtaining a degree is only the beginning of a long haul. The university course is a different ball game from the following years of general and specialist postgraduate training. Postgraduate training is physically, emotionally, and socially more demanding than the life of an undergraduate medical student on the one hand and of a settled doctor on the other. With so many uncertainties about tomorrow it is difficult to make secure and sensible decisions today. Be realistic, but do not falter simply for lack of courage; remember the words of Abraham Lincoln: "legs only have to be long enough to reach the ground".

This is your life; if you get it wrong you could become a square peg in a round hole or join the line of disillusioned dropouts. Like a submaster key, which opens both outer doors and a particular inner room, you need to fit both the necessary academic shape and also the required professional attitudes. In this new edition of *Learning Medicine* we give greater emphasis to the professionalism the public, and patients in particular, expect of their doctors and even of medical students. Finally, you need to dovetail into a particular speciality.

You must have the drive and ability to acquire a medical degree, equipping you to continue to learn on the job after that. Also, you need to be able to inspire trust and to accept that the interests of the patient come before the comfort or convenience of the doctor. It also helps a lot if you are challenged and excited by clinical practice. Personality, ability, and interest, shaped and shaved during the undergraduate course and the early postgraduate years, will fit you in due course, perhaps with a bit of a squeeze, into a particular speciality "hole". Sir James Paget, a famous London surgeon in the 19th century concluded from his 30 years of experience that the major determinant of students' success as doctors was "the personal character, the very nature, the will of each student".

Why do people want to become doctors? Medicine is a popular career choice for reasons perhaps both good and not so good. And who is to say whether the reasons for going in necessarily affect the quality of what comes out?

So, why medicine?

Glamour is not a good reason; television "soaps" and novels paint a false picture. The routine, repetitive, and tiresome aspects do not receive the prominence they deserve. On the other hand, the privilege (even if an inconvenience) of being on the spot when needed, of possessing the skill to make a correct diagnosis, and having the satisfaction of explaining, reassuring, and giving appropriate treatment can be immensely fulfilling even if demanding. Yet others who do not get their kicks that way might prefer a quieter life, and there is nothing wrong with that. It is a matter of horses for courses or, to return to the analogy, well-fitting pegs and holes.

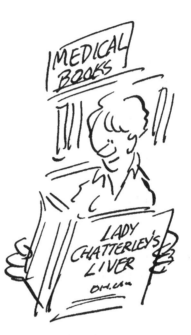

An interest in how the body works in health or in disease sometimes leads to a career in medicine. Such interest might, however, be equally well served by becoming an anatomist or physiologist and undertaking a lifetime study of the structure and function of the body. As for disease itself, many scientists study aspects of disease processes without having medical qualifications.

Many more people are curious about how the body works than either wish to or can become doctors. Nonetheless, for highly able individuals medicine does, as George Eliot wrote in *Middlemarch*, present "the most perfect interchange between science and art: offering the most direct alliance between intellectual conquest and the social good". Rightly or wrongly, it is not science itself which draws most people to medicine, but the amalgam of science and humanity.

Medical diagnosis is not like attaching a car engine to a computer. Accurate assessment of the outcome of a complex web of interactions of body, mind, and environment, which is the nature of much ill health, is not achieved that way. It is a far more subjective and judgmental process. Similarly, management of ill health is not purely mechanistic. It depends on a relationship of trust, a unique passport to the minds and bodies of all kinds and conditions of men, women, and children. In return the doctor has the ethical and practical duty to work uncompromisingly for the patient's interest. That is not always straightforward. One person's best interests may conflict with another's or with the interests of society as a whole – for example, through competition for limited or highly expensive treatment. On the other side of the coin, what is possible may not in fact be in the patient's best interest – for example, resuscitation in a hopeless situation in which the patient is unable to choose for him- or herself – leading to ethical dilemmas for the doctor and perhaps conflict with relatives.

Dedication to the needs of others is often given as a reason for wanting to be a doctor, but how do you either know or show you have it? Medicine has no monopoly on dedication but perhaps it is special because patients come first. As Sir Theodore Fox, for many years editor of the *Lancet*, put it:

> What is not negotiable is that our profession exists to serve the patient, whose interests come first. None but a saint could follow this principle all the time; but so many doctors have followed it so much of the time that the profession has been generally held in high regard. Whether its remedies worked or not, the public have seen medicine as a vocation, admirable because of a doctor's dedication.

A similar reason is a wish to help people, but policemen, porters, and plumbers do that too. If a more pastoral role is in mind why not become a priest, a social worker, or a schoolteacher? On the other hand, many are attracted by the special relationship between doctor and patient. This relationship of trust depends on the total honesty of the doctor. It has been said that, "Patients have a unique individual relationship with their doctors not encountered in any other profession and anything which undermines patients' confidence in that relationship will ultimately undermine the doctor's ability to carry out his or her work". A journalist writing in the *Sun* wrote cynically, "In truth there is not a single reason to suppose these days that doctors can be trusted any more than you can trust British Gas, a double glazing salesman, or the man in the pub". We disagree – and you would need to disagree too if you were to become a doctor. If it is of any comfort to the *Sun*, a Mori poll in 1999 asked a random selection of the public which professionals could be trusted to tell the truth. The results were: doctors 91%, judges 77%, scientists 63%, business leaders 28%, politicians 23%, and journalists 15%.

Professionalism includes the expectation that doctors (and medical students) can be relied on to look after their own health before taking responsibility for the care of others. Doctors who are heavy drinkers or users of prohibited drugs cannot guarantee the necessary clear and consistent judgement, quite apart from the undermining of trust through lawbreaking. Habits start young, and patients have a right to expect high standards of doctors and doctors in training, higher standards than society may demand of others.

Those not prepared for such personal discipline have an ethical duty not to choose medicine. It has been said that, "Trust is a very fragile thing: it can take years to build up; it takes seconds to destroy". Sir Thomas (later Lord) Bingham rejected an appeal to the Privy Council against the erasure of a doctor from the medical register, saying, "The reputation of the profession is more important than the fortunes of any individual member. Membership of a profession brings many benefits, but that is part of the price". The requirement for a doctor to be honest is stringent: at another Appeal against erasure in 1997, the Lord Justices of Appeal said, "This was a case in which the committee were entitled to take the view that the policy of preserving the public trust in the profession prevailed over strong mitigation; they were entitled to conclude … that there is no room for dishonest doctors".

The Hippocratic oath is essentially a commitment to absolute honesty, professional integrity, and being a good professional colleague. Many people feel that this spirit is so integral to being a doctor and should be so central to medical education and training that it does not need formal recitation on qualification, especially in the paternalistic phraseology of even modern versions of the Hippocratic oath. On the other hand is there not a place for a formal public declaration by new doctors of their explicit commitment to ethical conduct? Certainly the graduating medical students at many universities now make their own public statement affirming the principles of Good Medical Practice.

The General Medical Council (GMC) is not only responsible for maintaining a register of all doctors licensed to practise medicine in the UK but also for ensuring that doctors are trained to practise and do practise to a high standard. The GMC accepts that the public want to be looked after by doctors who are knowledgeable, skilful, honest, kind, and respectful of patients, and who do everything in their power to help them. Above all, that patients want a doctor they can trust. Explicit duties, responsibilities, values, and standards have been clearly set out on behalf of the profession by the

GMC in *Good Medical Practice*, which medical students now receive soon after arriving at medical school. (see Appendix 3) Now that contact with patients generally starts early in the course, so does the responsibility of medical students to be professional.

Medicine is an attractive career to good communicators and a difficult one for those who are not. The ability to develop empathy and understanding with all sorts of people in all sorts of situations is an important part of a doctor's art. It is part of medical training, but it helps greatly if it comes naturally in both speaking and writing. A sense of humour and broad interests also assist communication besides helping the doctor to survive as a person. Not all careers in medicine require face-to-face encounters with patients, but most require good teamwork with other doctors and health workers.

Arrogance, not unknown in the medical profession, hinders both good communication and teamwork. It is not justified: few doctors do things that others with similar training might not do as well, or better. Confidence based on competence and the ability to understand and cope is quite another matter; it is appreciated by patients and colleagues alike. Respect for others and an interest in and concern for their needs is essential. One applicant was getting near the point when she said at interview, "I like people", then paused and continued, "Well, I don't like them all, but I find them interesting". Patients can of course sometimes seem extremely demanding, difficult, unreasonable, and even hostile, particularly when you are exhausted.

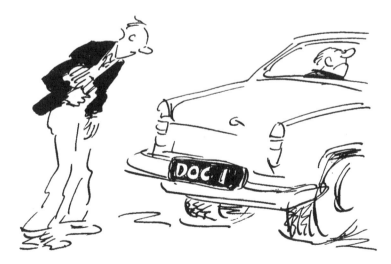

Many people consider medicine because they want to heal. Helping is more common than healing because much human illness is either incurable or will get better anyway. If curing is your main interest, better perhaps become a research pharmacologist developing new drugs. Also, bear in mind that the cost of attempting to cure, whether by drugs or by knife, is sometimes to make matters worse. A doctor must accept and honestly admit uncertainty and fallibility, inescapable parts of many occupations but harder to bear in matters of life and death.

Experience of illness near at hand, in oneself, friends, or family, may reinforce the desire to become a doctor. Having said that, the day-to-day detail of good care depends more on nurses than doctors and good career opportunities lie there too. In any event, the emotional impact of illness should be taken together with a broader perspective of the realities of the training and the opportunities and obligations of the career. Dr F. J. Inglefinger, editor of the *New England Journal of Medicine* wrote, when seriously ill himself:

In medical school, students are told about the perplexity, anxiety and misapprehension that may affect the patient … and in the clinical years the fortunate and sensitive student may learn much from talking to those assigned to his supervision. But the effects of lectures and conversations are ephemeral and are no substitute for actual experience. One might suggest, of course, that only those who have been hospitalised during their adolescent or adult years be admitted to medical school. Such a practice would not only increase the number of empathic doctors; it would also permit the whole elaborate system of medical school admissions to be jettisoned.

He had his tongue in his cheek, of course, but he also had his heart in his mouth.

Personal experience of the work and life of doctors, first and second hand, preferably in more than one of the different settings of general practice, hospital, or public health, is in any event formative and valuable in getting the feel of whether such work would suit. This can be difficult to arrange while you are still at school, not least because of the confidential nature of the doctor–patient relationship. Observation by a young person who may or may not eventually become a medical student is intrusive and requires great tact from the observer and good will from both doctor and patient. Doctors' children may have an advantage here (the only advantage they do have in the selection process) and could well be expected to know better than others what medical practice is all about. Most applicants have to make do with seeing medicine from another side by helping in hospital, nursing home, or general practitioner's (GP's) surgery, each situation giving different insights.

And, why not?

Learning medicine involves an education and training longer and more disruptive of personal life than in any other profession. And medicine is moving so fast that doctors can never stop learning. To be trained, it is said, is to have arrived; to be educated is still to be travelling.

Unsocial hours of work are almost inevitable for students and junior doctors, and are a continuing obligation in many specialities. If this really is not how you are prepared to spend your life, better not to start than to complain or drop out later. That does not, however, mean that the profession and public has any excuse for failing to press for improvements in working conditions of all doctors, especially for those in training. Exhausted doctors are neither good nor safe, and it becomes difficult for them to profit fully from the lessons of their experience.

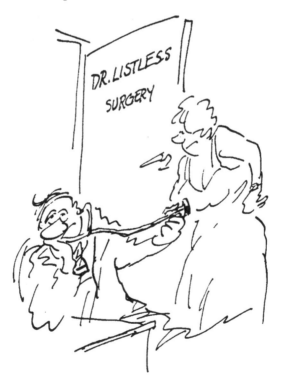

What about medicine for a good salary, security, social position, and a job which can in theory be done anywhere? Doctors in the UK are paid poorly in comparison with other doctors in Western Europe, North America, and Australasia, unless they supplement their income with a busy private practice, but, having said that, the pay is not bad. It became clear over the millennium that the UK had for many years been training fewer doctors than it needed. As a result there has recently been a substantial increase in the number of medical students in the UK but, almost simultaneously, the NHS has been reducing the number of posts for trained doctors. Suddenly, and we hope temporarily, medicine has become a less secure profession.

Social advancement would also be a poor motive for entering medicine, unlikely to achieve its aim. The profession has largely been knocked off its traditional pedestal. Much of the mystery of medicine has been dispelled by good scientific writing and television. Public confidence has been eroded by critical reports of error and incompetence, not to mention a rising tide of litigation against doctors. In the words of Sir Donald Irvine, Former President of the GMC: "The public expectation of doctors is changing. Today's patients are better informed. They expect their doctors to behave properly and to perform consistently well, and are less tolerant of poor practice". Such respect that doctors still enjoy has to be continually earned by high standards of professionalism.

The freedom of doctors to practise in other countries is no longer what it was. Most developed countries have restrictions on doctors trained elsewhere. European Union countries are open to UK doctors but none is short of doctors, and language barriers have to be overcome. Need and opportunity still exist in developing countries. All in all, there are less demanding ways than medicine of making a good living and having the opportunity to work abroad.

Making your own decision

It would be pompous and old fashioned to insist that all medical students should have a vocation but they do need to be prepared to put themselves out, to *earn* respect, to impose self-discipline, and to take the rough with the smooth in their training and career; they also need to be excited and challenged intellectually and emotionally by some if not all aspects of medicine.

And, as much of the decision-making in medicine is made on incomplete evidence, they must be able to live with uncertainty. They also need the necessary patience and determination to improve imperfect treatment, increasingly practising "evidence-based" medicine.

It is neither necessary nor normal for individuals to be entirely clear why they want to become a doctor. Those who think they do and also know precisely the sort of doctor they want to be usually change their minds more than once during their training. Whatever your reasons for medicine, the first thing to do is to test your interest as best you can against what the career involves, its demands, its privileges, and its responsibilities. It is not useful to try to decide now what sort of doctor you might want to be, in fact you do not need to decide for at least 7 years. But it is wise towards the end of the undergraduate course to examine speciality career options more carefully than most students do now, not least so that enthusiasm about the possibility of a particular specialist career can help motivate you through finals and especially through the somewhat harrowing clinical responsibility of the early postgraduate years.

At the end of the day, your decisions must be your own. If you have questions about course or career, find out who to ask and make your own enquiries; it is your life and your responsibility to make a suitable career choice. Do not let your parents, however willing or however wise, choose your career for you. Beware the fate of Dr Blifil in *Tom Jones* who was described as:

… a gentleman who had the misfortune of losing the advantage of great talents by the obstinacy of his father, who would breed him for a profession he disliked … the doctor had been obliged to study physick [medicine], or rather to say that he had studied it …

The trust of others, regardless of wealth, poverty, or position, together with the opportunity to understand, explain, and care, if not cure, can bring great fulfilment. So too can the challenge of pushing back the frontiers of medical science and of improving medical practice.

Medicine requires a lively mind, wise judgment, sharp eyes, perceptive hearing, a stout heart, a steady hand, and the ability to learn continuously. It is an ideal career for all rounders and the better rounded you are the wider your career opportunity in medicine as clinician, scientist, teacher, researcher, journalist, or even politician.

Medicine will never be an entirely comfortable or convenient career. It also requires signing up to an ethical code stronger than the law of the land and, even as a student, observing the law – high spirits notwithstanding. Doctors' convictions are never spent. Doctors breaching the law or their ethical code may lose their registration, their licence to practise, and with that their livelihood.

The configuration of an individual's character, aspirations, and abilities have to match the shape of the opportunity, like pegs in holes. Becoming and being a doctor is not by any means everyone's cup of tea. Yet for all its demands, medicine offers a deeply satisfying and rewarding lifetime of service to those prepared to give themselves to it.

REMEMBER

- Becoming a doctor takes 5 or 6 years.

- Further postgraduate training takes about as long again.

- There is much to be said both for and against a career in medicine.

- Discover as much as possible about what being a doctor involves before making a decision which will affect the rest of your life.

- Try spending time talking to medical students, hospital doctors, or local GPs.

- The decision for or against applying to medical school should be your own – do not be pressured by school, parents, or friends – it is your life.

2

Opportunity and reality

Statistically, the chances of entry to medical school are pretty good: currently approximately 19,000 home, European Union (EU), and overseas applicants compete for nearly 8000 places to read medicine at UK universities. Since 2000, moves by the Government to increase the numbers of doctors in the NHS have prompted a surge of 2000 new places to read medicine in the UK.

In his report, *Learning from Bristol* (2001), Prof. Sir Ian Kennedy recommended that:

Access to medical schools should be widened to include people from diverse academic and socio-economic backgrounds. Those with qualifications in other areas of health care and those with educational background in subjects other than science, who have the ability and wish to, should have greater opportunities than is presently the case, to enter medical school.

In fact, most medical schools will consider applicants without a strong science background, especially for some graduate entry courses.

Most applicants come from professional or clerical backgrounds. Many others still see medicine as a closed shop in which, if you do not have such a background, you stand little chance of either entry or success. On the contrary, research has shown that once academic ability has been discounted neither social class, age, medical relatives, nor type of secondary school affect chances of entry to medical school. But examination results depend partly on educational opportunity at school, not to mention encouragement to study at home. Many medical schools try to take educational opportunity into account.

The fact of the matter is that many people simply do not believe they have a real opportunity to become a doctor. Many who might well make excellent doctors and would broaden the perspectives and insights of the medical profession as a whole simply do not apply. If they do not apply, they cannot be considered.

Academic achievement is the most important determinant of success in selection. Some medical schools make their final selection on grades alone; most also take account of attitudes, personality, and broader achievements, qualities which being difficult to measure require judgment to assess and therefore cannot be proved to be absolutely fair. Nevertheless, an immense amount of effort is put into making selection as fair as possible.

The long course of study, diminishing educational grants, mounting student debts, and course fees also tend to deter those without financial backing. It is extremely difficult to work one's way through medical school. Spare time jobs are difficult to find, and the course leaves little time for them, especially in the later years with on call duties in hospital. The fact that the job is secure at the end of the road and is sufficiently well paid for debts to be repaid seems just too far away to be any consolation.

Opportunities for women

Universities across the world were slow to give women equal opportunity to higher education, and medicine was perhaps the slowest professional course of all. Several UK medical schools first admitted women as students only 56 years ago (except during the world wars when they were unable to fill all their places with men).

Women now have equal opportunity to enter medicine. In 1991, for the first time, more women than men were admitted to medical school in the UK, and the following year, for the first time women predominated among both applicants and entrants. This trend continues, and in 2006 the proportions of women and men in both applications and entrants was about 56% women and 44% men. Such is the turn around of the imbalance of men and women students that some admissions tutors are asking if the time has come to consider ways of encouraging male applicants, although there is as yet no talk of quotas or positive action for men!

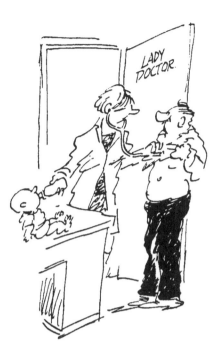

Although it can still be argued that the medical profession as a whole is still male dominated, there is no doubt that as the trend towards more women students continues, this is being slowly but surely broken down by sheer force of the numbers of women doctors. Some specialities remain more challenging for women to succeed in than others, but some fields are naturally finding the majority of their new recruits are women.

In the past, careers advisers, parents, and applicants were understandably aware of the potential personal conflicts ahead between career and family at a time when, even more than today, women were left holding the baby while the man got on with his career. Times have changed, and society's attitudes to parenting are changing all the time. Also the conflict between career and personal interests is not confined to women and to bringing up a family. Some argue positively for medicine as being better placed than many other careers for resolving this conflict, as Dr Susan Andrew has done:

Medicine is a most suitable career for intelligent, educated women who aspire to married life, because it carries far more opportunities for flexible working than other professions … My message is: remember, women have struggled for centuries to have lives of their own and to be defined in terms of their own achievements, not someone else's.

Ethnic minorities

Medicine, science, and engineering are all disproportionately popular university courses with home students from ethnic minorities, especially those of Indian or southeast Asian origin. More than a quarter of home applicants to medical school are drawn from ethnic minorities, although they comprise less than one-tenth of the UK population. Afro-Caribbeans are an exception, reflecting their current general academic underachievement, a cause of national concern; medical schools are keen to encourage them to apply.

Concern has also been expressed that applicants from ethnic minorities with equivalent academic grades were found a few years ago to be less likely to be shortlisted for interview; once interviewed, however, they were as likely to receive an offer as anyone else. The difference was small, less than the disadvantage at that time of applying towards the end of the application period, but it still existed in a survey in 1998. One reason may be that these applicants have had less opportunity and encouragement to develop leadership skills, to pursue wider interests, and to participate in community service, all important dimensions at shortlisting in most medical schools. Prejudice may also have been a factor because a similar disadvantage has been found in shortlisting for junior hospital posts. A study a few years ago showed that when identical curriculum vitae (CVs) were submitted under different names, those bearing a European name were more likely to be shortlisted than others for senior house officer posts. Since 1998 stringent steps have been taken in all medical schools to ensure equal opportunities, and no recent evidence has caused concern.

A small but significant minority of Indian or Asian women students experience family pressures which undermine their ability to cope happily or effectively with their academic work. Parents and grandparents may curtail freedom, command frequent presence (a demand not limited to the women students or indeed to Asian families), and occasionally impose arranged marriages. Deans are familiar with situations in which they have to send down students for academic failure due to such pressures. Parents must better understand that until the pressures that are preventing their child from working effectively are removed, by giving them more personal and intellectual liberty, they have no prospect of being readmitted to a medical course.

Of course, families of any section of society can place pressures on a student, such as a young student who has to care for younger siblings or an elderly relative. While these pressures are understandable, and often, inadvertent, can it ever be acceptable to undermine a young person's chances in life, however difficult the family circumstances?

Mature students

Age is statistically no disadvantage in application to medical school, but until recently that may well have been because few mature students have had the necessary academic and financial credentials to apply. The encouragement of the development of fast-track courses specifically for graduates has greatly improved the opportunity for mature students in medicine (see p. 60). Not all mature entrants to medicine are graduates but they have to apply to the standard course. Most medical schools welcome the contribution mature students make to the stability and responsibility of their year group and more widely within the medical school as a result of their greater experience, achievement, and sensitivity. Maturity helps in communication and empathy with patients, to the extent that many deans would prefer to take all their students over the age of 21 years. This acceptance is reflected by statistics – since 2000 the proportion of mature students applying to and entering undergraduate medicine has almost doubled. In 2005 the percentage of mature medical students (aged 25 or over at year of entry) reached 10% of the total.

Good organisation, a sufficient income, and an understanding partner with a flexible job (if any partner at all) are the foundations of successful medical study by mature students with family responsibilities. The early years of the course are no more difficult for medicine than other degree courses, except in that the intensity of lectures and practical work is greater than in most other subjects. Efficient use of time during the day and a regular hour or two of study most evenings (with more before examinations) should suffice. Some students manage to support themselves for a year or two by evening and weekend jobs. It is not easy and becomes more or less impossible during the later years, when the working year is 48 weeks. Most clinical assignments require one night or weekend in hospital every week or two. Two or three "residences" – for example, in obstetrics or paediatrics – may require living in a distant hospital for a week or two at a time, learning as one of the medical team by day and sometimes at night. An increasing

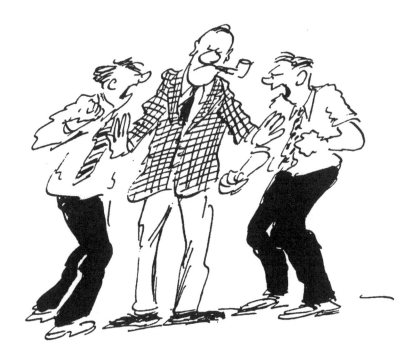

number of schools send their students to district hospitals often some miles from the university town, for much longer periods of time than before. If this is likely to cause major problems with some students it is worth checking this out before you choose where to apply. The working day at that stage is long, starting at 8.00 am and finishing about 5.00 pm or later, with most weekends free. The elective period of 2 or 3 months is often spent abroad but may be spent close to home and does not necessarily entail night or weekend duty. Finally, several weeks as a shadow house officer involves residence in hospital at the end of the course.

Some mature students manage magnificently. One who started just over the age of 30 and had two children aged between 5 and 10 and a husband willing and able to adjust his working hours to hers had studied for A levels when she was a busy mother. Her further education college described her as the most academically and personally outstanding student that they could remember; she won several prizes on her way through medical school and qualified without difficulty. Another of similar age with four children and separated from her husband coped with such amazing energy and effectiveness, despite considerable financial hardship (and the help of a succession of competent and reliable au pairs) that she left everyone breathless. Exceptional these two may be, but it can be done, requiring as Susan Spindler commented in her book, *Doctors to Be*, "an unerring sense of priorities in her life, tremendous stamina and the capacity to concentrate briefly but hard".

Mature students are at a substantial financial disadvantage if they have already had a student loan for higher education. Even if eligible for bursaries or additional loans, those who have already achieved financial independence find their reduced circumstances tough.

Finance is only one of the problems facing mature students: to revert from being an independent individual to becoming one of a bunch of recent school leavers can be both hard and tiresome, although most mature students in medicine seem to cope with this transition remarkably well. Shorter courses (4 years) for some graduates have now been introduced at several universities, with students supported for the last 3 years by NHS bursaries (see p. 57). Better let a mature student, an Oxford graduate in psychology, give her own impressions:

The mature student's tale

I have always felt that the term "mature student" is vaguely uncomplimentary – almost synonymous with "fuddy old fart" or "bearded hippy". Personally I have never considered myself particularly "mature" in comparison with my year group, while others merely describe themselves as being slightly less immature. Some of us have had previous jobs ranging from city slicker to nurse or army officer, while others may have come straight from a previous degree or are supporting a family. Whatever the difference in background one common factor unites us all, we are convinced that medicine is now the career for us. Deciding this a little later than most brings its own particular problems.

To start with, the interview tends to be rather different to that of a school leaver. There are usually only three questions that the panel really want answering. Firstly, why did you decide to study medicine now? Is it a realistic decision, or just a diversion from a midlife crisis, do you know what the job actually entails, and how can you assure them you will not change your mind again? Secondly, "How do you think you will cope being *so* much older than everybody else", which I found rather patronising, but it is wise to have thought of a suitable response. Thirdly, and most importantly, how will you finance yourself? No medical school wants to give a place to someone who will subsequently drop out due to financial pressure.

Most mature medical students undoubtedly find that the financial burden poses the biggest problem. While it is possible to finance yourself through scholarships, charities, loans, and overdrafts, this takes a lot of time and organisation. Most medical schools still want a financial guarantor in addition. Many students get a part-time job to ease the pressure but during a heavily timetabled and examined medical course this can prove difficult. Progression through to the clinical years brings even fewer opportunities for work with unpredictable hours and scarce holidays. It is worth investigating which medical schools and universities are more accepting of mature students, and which have funds to help financially. Aside from the obvious practical problems of having little money, coping with the financial divide between yourself and old friends now earning can take some getting used to.

Once the financial issues have been hurdled, other worries surface. Fitting in with school leavers may initially be viewed as a problem, but if you can survive Freshers' Week I can assure you it does get easier. Progressing through the course, the proportion of shared experience increases and the initial age and experience gap no longer poses such a problem. One particular advantage of the length of the medical course is that those in the final year may be of a similar age to those entering as mature students, and due to the wide range of clubs and societies offered by most universities there is ample opportunity to meet people of all ages.

One advantage of being that little bit older is that it is much easier not to feel you have to succumb to the peer group pressure so often prevalent in the medical school environment. When faced with the tempting offer to stand naked on a table and down a yard of ale, the excuse "I've got to get home to the wife and kids" will usually suffice. The attitude of some medical students to those older than themselves can occasionally be somewhat disconcerting. A first-year student was recently heard to comment to a mature student in her year, "Isn't it funny, you are in our year, but when we come back for reunions, you will probably be dead".

A variety of roles may be created by your new peer group for you to fit in to. These can range from being initially seen as the "old freak" or "year swot" to pseudo parent or agony aunt. These roles do tend to diminish over time, and most mature students are viewed as an asset as they bring in a different range of knowledge and experience. The importance of maintaining old friendships and having an outlet away from medicine, however, cannot be overemphasised.

"Will I be able to cope with the work?" can obviously be a further worry. A levels may seem a dim and distant memory, and the type of work or learning most mature students have been previously doing is a far cry from the vast amounts of memorising required by the medical course. There is no doubt about it – studying medicine is a lot of work, with regular examinations and a full timetable. Most mature students do seem to have developed a better notion of time management and efficient learning, however, and this, coupled with a strong motivation to complete the course, can alleviate some of the work pressure.

Being a clinical student learning on the wards brings its own particular problems. The transition from having a respected job or being an instrumental part of a team to having no exact role perhaps presents more difficulties to a mature student than to others. The unpleasant "teaching by humiliation" method employed by some doctors may be particularly trying to mature students, especially when (as has been known to happen) the person being so patronising was in your little sister's year at school. Being at the very bottom of such an entrenched hierarchy can be wearing and frustrating. Overall, however, most doctors involved in teaching are extremely supportive of mature students, and a proportion feel all medical students should gain outside experience before embarking on a medical career.

Progressing through the training the clinical aspects of the course become more important and, for the majority of students, more enjoyable. Mature students tend to find this especially true and are often in a position of strength, being more confident and relaxed in their interactions with patients, bringing skills and experience from previous careers. Personally I have found this is one of the greatest assets of being a mature student, finding emotional or difficult situations easier to cope with than if I had come straight into medicine from school.

The downside can be that fellow students and doctors can have a higher expectation of your abilities and knowledge. While this may be true in some aspects of communication, the learning curve for practical skills is just the same as for others. Being a few years older does not necessarily mean you are an instant pro at inserting a catheter.

Once you have realistically decided that medicine is the career for you, possibly sat required A levels, got through the interview, and faced up to the prospect of at least 5 years' financial hardship, is it all worth it?

Being a mature student it is all the more important to make sure that the decision to study medicine is not viewed idealistically. There are some doctors who deeply regret the decision to go into the profession. One doctor, who was a mature student, replied when asked, "It was the worst decision I ever made. I'm permanently tired and just don't have the time I would like for myself or family anymore".

Older students obviously often have different commitments and priorities which their younger colleagues are yet to experience, such as children or a mortgage. While life through medical school can be hard, with academic stress and financial worry, difficulties do not end with qualification. Becoming a doctor not only brings new opportunities but also a different way of life. The line between work and personal life can become increasingly blurred. Despite a more enlightened approach to junior doctors' hours, the time commitment is still immense. The work ethic is unlike that of any other career. This means that inevitable sacrifices have to be made in one's personal life, and consideration as to how this will affect present or future partners and children is important.

Having stated many of the difficulties, the advantages of being a mature student are considerable. Medicine, perhaps more than any other profession, requires a maturity of insight, both personally and in dealing with patients; many situations are emotionally demanding and stressful; coping with added academic pressure can be tiring and demoralising. A more mature approach together with a greater certainty in your career choice is a definite asset. Maintaining friendships outside medicine means that when it all gets a bit too much you can escape, and being offered a second chance at being a student can mean you make far more of the opportunities offered to you than when you first left school. Overall I have found medicine to be fascinating and enjoyable. The career choices available once you are in the profession are extremely varied so finding your niche should be possible. The combination of human contact with academic interest is unlike that of any other career, and the unique privilege of being so intimately involved in people's lives never fails to be exciting or interesting. It is possible and personally I feel it is worth it ... (but ask me again when I'm a junior doctor).

SE

Overseas applicants

About 2300 overseas students compete for about 550 places. Fast-track courses and the standard courses in the newest medical schools (Brighton/Sussex, Hull-York, Peninsula, and University of East Anglia), set up specifically to address the shortage of doctors in the NHS, are not open to overseas students. Overseas students are liable for full fees, amounting to a total of about £70,000 over 5 years. They will also need about £50,000 for their living expenses. It is no longer possible for someone from overseas to be classified as a home student by purchasing secondary education at a British school, by nominating a "guardian" with a UK address, or by buying a UK residence. Nor are British expatriates working permanently abroad normally eligible for home fee status.

Local education authorities (LEA) are responsible for finally determining fee status; the guidelines state that students are able to pay fees at the home rate only if they have been "ordinarily resident" in the UK or in a member state of the EU in the previous 3 years and have not been resident during any part of that period wholly or mainly for the purpose of receiving full-time education. Exception is made for nationals or their children who have not been ordinarily resident during that period because of temporary employment abroad. Officially recognised refugees and people granted asylum or exceptional leave to remain in the UK are also treated as exceptions.

Overseas students are entitled to stay for 4 years and sometimes longer after graduation to undertake their specialist postgraduate medical education in the UK, in which capacity they make a welcome contribution as junior doctors.

Equal opportunities, equal difficulties?

Opportunity to enter medicine has, as far as can be judged, become equal for those realistic about their qualifications. But everyone considering becoming a doctor must look behind and beyond medical school to the reality of whether a career in medicine is for them a pathway to fulfilment or to frustration. The tension between the relative freedom of many careers and the ties of medicine face men and women alike. But medicine is a tougher career for many women than for most men. A few years ago we received a letter from three students from St George's Hospital Medical School in London, indignant about the suggestion that the position of women requires special consideration: "For a start, let's bury the idea that male and female students have different aspirations – we all wish to end up well rounded human beings ..." Sure, but it is not necessary to become a doctor to do that, although medical education will have failed in part of its purpose if all doctors are not "well-rounded" individuals.

The difficulties particularly facing women doctors are both subtle and unsubtle. The obvious are the dual responsibilities of family and career, which most women do not wish to know about, consider, or even recognise when they are medical students but which they begin to come to terms with once the all consuming task of qualifying as a doctor has been achieved. Opportunities for part-time training and employment in many specialities are limited. Career dice are loaded against those who patiently plod through long years of part-time training. Progress towards a training and a career structure which would fully harness skills of (in future) at least half the medical workforce is slow. The personal and national cost of failure to use the skills of women doctors fully would be immense.

The potential disadvantages for women in postgraduate training can be and often are overcome supremely well with good family support. Recent changes in taxation allowances also mean better financial support for working families through tax relief on childcare. Some specialities – such as general practice, pathology, radiology, anaesthetics, and public health – can readily be made flexible and compatible with other responsibilities.

The more subtle difficulties facing women include the feeling that more is demanded of them as doctors because they are women. Not all women agree but a woman doctor, Fran Reichenberg, wrote that:

Both patients and staff expect far more of female doctors. These expectations arise from traditional female roles in society of mother, carer, so other of the distressed …

She also believed that male doctors may get special treatment from the team:

The perks of the male house officer who shows a clear interest in the female staff include his intravenous fluids being drawn up and done, his results filed for him, his blood forms filled out. Many telephone calls chasing results being done for him. … These differences amount to many extra hours' work a week for the female house officer and exacerbate her fatigue and low morale.

In our experience, special treatment can work both ways.

Women compete very effectively but sometimes against the odds. The unsaid concern about the organisational and financial impact of maternity leave seems to confer no overall disadvantage. Women may, however, suffer disproportionately from the innate conservatism of consultant appointments committees. Most members of appointments committees and most remaining consultants in post are for historical reasons men. Having more women on appointments committees is not necessarily the answer: on one occasion the strongest opposition to taking gender into account in appointing to an obstetric team serving an ethnic population with substantial preferences for women doctors came from the only woman on the committee.

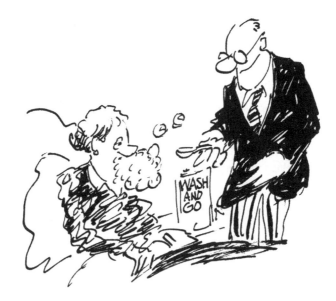

Many women still feel at a disadvantage, as Dr Anne Nicol, a consultant pathologist, explained:

Unless we remove the glass ceiling, many top candidates for consultant posts will fail to reach the top. Let's face it, jobs go to the applicant wanted by the consultants in post … [who] still see the ideal colleague as someone much like themselves … you can almost hear them say "one has to be able to get on with him – he has to be on your wave length"… tribalism among male consultants is strong, pressure to be one of the herd intense; Tory voting, middle class, privately educated, golf playing white males are the tribal group most likely to succeed …

The common perception is that women don't fit in, are difficult to work with and can never be one of the tribe. A woman making a vocal stance on a topic will find it is not long before someone comments on her hormonal balance or time of month …

We can ensure that more women at least get their noses pressed against the glass ceiling by creating more family-friendly training packages, part-time posts and job shares.

Each aspiring entrant to medicine must come to terms with the length and the nature of the training, the demands of the career, and the reality of his or her own personality and ability. Add to this a strategic view of the opportunity – open and equal on merit at the beginning, convoluted later for several reasons, but destined to become more equal. Finally, the professional responsibility of putting patients first is inescapable, often uncomfortable, but fulfilling.

REMEMBER

- Anyone with ability and aptitude stands a chance of admission to medical school; background does not matter.

- Once academic achievement has been taken into account, social class, age, having parents who are doctors, or the type of school you attended will not affect your chances of admission.

- Being a woman gives a slight but statistically significant increase in your chances.

- Mature students are welcomed by most medical schools but they often have to overcome both financial and personal difficulties; fast-track courses are available to graduates.

- Students with children will need good home support.

- About 2300 overseas students apply for 550 places reserved for them at UK medical schools.

3

Requirements for entry

Entry to medical school is academically the most competitive moment in the student's life. However, becoming a doctor requires many more qualities than brain power, including compassion, endurance, determination, communication skills, enthusiasm, intellectual curiosity, balance, adaptability, integrity, and a sense of humour. All these are highly desirable attributes but not absolute "requirements" for entry to medicine: few have them all but a remarkable number of applicants have many.

Academic ability is an essential requirement for entry, and the ability to pass examinations remains important throughout the course and the subsequent years of postgraduate training. Less competitive than A levels, but no less intense, were the traditional end of first and second year examinations on the sciences underpinning medicine. New curricula that emphasise understanding and integration of knowledge rather than "facts" are tested more by continuous assessment, a less destructive process than a series of annual crises but not without a constantly recurring academic tension. Professionally, the hardest examinations are those for the higher specialist diplomas of fellowship or membership of the Medical Royal Colleges, requiring a broad and solid grasp of the clinical skills, knowledge, and, to an increasing extent, the attitudes appropriate to a specialist. "Finals" – the examinations for the Bachelor of Medicine and Surgery degree, the degree which acts as the basis for a provisional licence to practise as a doctor, are largely a matter of hard slog, particularly in the later years. They used to be taken as a big bang at the end of the course but are now broken up at most universities over a period of about 18 months.

Broader requirements

Although all doctors need to be bright (not less perhaps than what it takes to get three B grades at A level at first attempt), medicine needs a great deal more than academic ability. Applicants must not forget that chances of success in the admissions process rest as much on additional skills – ability to communicate, empathy and integrity – as they do on academic prowess. Any admissions tutor will be looking to assess your awareness of the qualities that any good doctor requires. Dr Phillip Hay of St George's summarises these attributes as:

• knowledge and understanding
• proficiency in basic clinical skills
• attitudes necessary for good medical practice and patient care
• intellectual curiosity and critical skills
• good teamwork
• lifelong learning
• robustness
• thoroughness
• awareness of own limitations
• open-mindedness
• reflectiveness
• cultural awareness
• sensitivity to life-cycle changes.

The only way of achieving such awareness is work experience. Whether you volunteer in a nursing home, shadow your local GP, visit a hospital and talk to staff, or care for an elderly or disabled relative, you should come away with a clear and realistic perspective of what illness can mean for patient and for doctor.

For more information on volunteering and practical experience, see the list of addresses in Appendix 4.

The ability to communicate well, to work in a team with a confident but not arrogant manner, and to be prepared as need arises to lead and take responsibility is important too. A sense of humour sprinkles oil on the wheels of communication.

Endurance, determination, and perseverance are part of the same package. They feed on dual enthusiasm for science and for the healing art of medicine.

They are inspired by curiosity and enriched by sparks of initiative and originality. Lord Moran (Dean of St Mary's and Winston Churchill's doctor) once said, "The student who is not curious is surely no student at all; he is already old, and his thoughts are borrowed thoughts".

Becoming a doctor is not as formidable as it sounds, given good friends, teachers, and opportunities to learn, but it requires solid organisation of time and life and being self-propelled. Desirable characteristics for medicine do not end here. Balance is needed; balance which comes from an intellectual and personal life is broader and deeper than academic success alone. Prof. David Greenfield, first Dean of the University of Nottingham Medical School, referred to "balance of scientific and clinical excellence, humanitarian and compassionate concern … balance of service and learning, balance of current competence and future adaptability". Other interests – literary, musical, artistic, and sporting – encourage achievement, provide recreation, and demand application, enthusiasm, and ability. They can become great stabilisers and good points of communication with both colleagues and

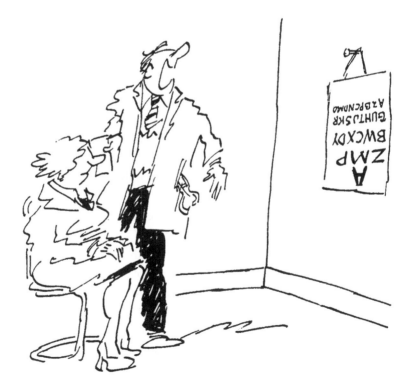

patients. For a female accident and emergency consultant, to also be the medical officer for a well-known football club (not that she is a great player) is good for her and for her hospital.

Then there is the invaluable down-to-earth ability to organise and to cope; a capable pair of hands and a reassuring attitude of "leave it to me and I'll sort it out", taking huge weights off shoulders and loads off minds. Sir George Pickering, one-time Regius Professor of Medicine at Oxford, wrote, "Medicine is in some ways the most personal and responsible profession: the patient entrusts his life and wellbeing to his doctor. Thus, the character and personality of the doctor, his sympathy and understanding, his sense of responsibility, his selflessness are as important as his scientific and technical knowledge". He also pointed out that a doctor neither needs to nor should try to sort out every problem him or herself: "the best doctors know to whom to turn for help".

Many medical schools, when asked which qualities they regarded as most important in applicants to medicine, highlighted the desirability of a realistic understanding of what is demanded in the study of medicine and in the subsequent career. Without this embryo insight, many years of unhappiness may lie ahead, however bright and however gifted the student. Failure to understand the demands of the job and the limitations of the art may explain why some doctors drop out of medicine.

Applicants from medical backgrounds have an advantage in this respect. They have seen the effects of the career on their parents and families, and have had the opportunity to explore what their parent or parents do; they also have relatively easy access to observing other medical specialities. All the more regrettable if they have not taken this opportunity to find out what it is all about. For others, it is much more difficult. Most television medical programmes glamorise and trivialise, and give little insight into the everyday undramatic life of a doctor. The BBC TV series *Doctors to Be* and *Doctors At Large*, following students through their years at St Mary's, and now for 20 years into their careers, are an exception and offer useful insights, even if the structure of the course itself has now changed. The rather embattled and disillusioned group of new doctors at the end of the first series has now been balanced by glimpses of where they are now, 10 years on, and reveals that they feel that it has all been worthwhile. A 20-year follow-up is now in preparation. As this is one of the most fundamental aspects of making an informed personal decision *Learning Medicine* puts less emphasis on the years in medical school and more on where they lead.

Personal health requirements and disability

A doctor's overriding responsibility is the safety and well-being of patients. As such all applicants to medical school must have the potential to function as a fully competent doctor and fulfil the rigorous demands of professional fitness to practise as stated by the General Medical Council. All applicants must therefore disclose any disabilities or medical conditions on the application form as they may affect the ability to practise medicine. This may be by placing patients at risk of infection, being unable to perform necessary medical procedures, or by impairing your judgement. Similarly, applicants must also complete a declaration that they have no criminal convictions or pending prosecutions, in line with national policies for staff working in sensitive roles. In most circumstances a declaration does not automatically disqualify an applicant but will allow the case to be decided on its own merits.

The UK Department of Health has requirements for specific conditions, which means that a student cannot be admitted with active tuberculosis or if infectious with hepatitis B, until they can be proven to be no longer infectious. In the case of hepatitis B, all prospective students must show proof of adequate immunisation before commencing the course. You will be asked for documentary proof when you arrive at medical school. Your own general practitioner (GP) can usually arrange for hepatitis B immunisation to be carried out. The course and testing for a satisfactory response can take up to 9 months, so you should discuss this with your GP at the earliest opportunity. If there is a failure to respond to the immunisation a student will be expected to prove that they are not infectious. In these rare circumstances, or where a student tests positive for any of the hepatitis B antigens, they should discuss this with their GP and the admissions tutor of their preferred school, as soon as possible.

There is no clear national policy as yet about candidates who are known to be hepatitis C positive. However, this must be declared on the UCAS form, and individual schools will advise in this rare instance. In any event, failure to disclose any condition that puts patients at risk will result in immediate dismissal from medical school.

All students are advised to be immunised against meningococcal meningitis before starting at university.

Any disability should also be disclosed and will be dealt with by the schools on a case-by-case basis. Dyslexia should also be disclosed on the UCAS form and this will need to be supported by a formal statement from a suitably qualified psychologist. Most medical schools will advise relevant departments of the assistance which may be necessary for students with dyslexia and will make some time allowances in written examinations, but no concessions are made in clinical examinations.

Taking illegal drugs or abusing alcohol are also inconsistent with a doctor's professional responsibilities, both on patient safety grounds and the need for personal integrity. Students who ignore their responsibility to be utterly dependable in this regard put their place in medical school in severe jeopardy.

Academic requirements

Although academic achievement is only the qualifying standard for entering the real field of selection, like the Olympic qualifying standard is to selection for the national team, it is overwhelmingly the strongest element in selection. Unlike all the other desirable attributes of personality, attitude, and interest examination results look deceptively objective. Relatively objective they may be but they are still poor indicators of the potential to become "a good doctor" – a product difficult to define, not least because medicine is such a wide career that there may be many different sorts of good doctors – but they all need the appropriate knowledge, skills, and attitudes for effective medical practice and the ability to use them competently.

Examination results at the age of 18 years do not predict late developers nor do they take account of differences in educational opportunity at school nor of support for study at home. Results may also be upset by ill health on the day; even minor illness or discomfort crucially timed may take the gloss off the performance, a gloss which may make all the difference between a place at medical school and no place at all. Having said that, however, those who fail during the medical course are generally those with the poorest A level results, and those who do best, especially in the early years with their greater scientific content, are generally those with the highest. But there are outstanding exceptions.

All medical schools set a minimum standard of at least AAB at A level (Table 3.1 and 3.2). The actual achievement of entrants is very similar at all universities whatever their target requirements, except Oxford and Cambridge, where they are higher. Medical schools which set marginally lower grades leave themselves the flexibility to make allowances for special situations and to give due weight to outstanding non-academic attributes. Most successful applicants to medical schools setting a lower minimum substantially exceed their requirements. It is vital to realise that good grades do not guarantee a place: far more applicants achieve the necessary grades than can be given a place.

Chemistry or physical science is required by all universities for medicine. They prefer this at A level, but practically all of the medical schools in the UK are prepared to accept AS chemistry in place of A level. Most are prepared to accept a combination of AS levels in place of another science or mathematics A level. In practice, AS levels are normally offered in addition to three A levels and not in substitution for one. Many universities prefer two other science subjects at A level, taken from the group of physics (unless physical science is offered), biology, and mathematics, but all are prepared to accept a good grade in an arts subject in place of one, or in some medical schools, two science subjects. Some medical schools do not accept mathematics and higher mathematics together as two of the required three A level subjects. General studies A level is generally not acceptable as one of the subjects.

All medical schools are prepared to accept one and sometimes more than one non-science or mathematics A level.

No particular non-science subjects are favoured but knowledge-based rather than practical skills-based subjects are generally preferred. It may be difficult to compare grades in arts and science subjects, so a higher target may be set for an arts subject for entry to medicine. Several universities express a preference for biology over physics or mathematics. Chemistry and biology are the foundations of medical science, especially if the mathematical aspects of those subjects are included. But however useful it is to be numerate in medicine, especially in research, students without a good knowledge of biology find themselves handicapped at least in the first year of the course by their lack of understanding of cell and organ function and its terminology. They also generally have greater difficulty in expressing themselves in writing, especially if their first language is not English. Failure

Table 3.1. For applicants with qualifications from England, Wales and Northern Ireland

University	GCE entry requirements	A levels	AS levels	Other Info
Aberdeen	AAB	Acceptable on its own and combined with other qualifications. Chemistry is highly desirable, plus at least one from Biology, Mathematics or Physics and one other. General Studies excluded.	Acceptable only when combined with other qualifications. General Studies excluded.	UKCAT compulsory
Barts, London, Queen Mary	AAB	Acceptable on its own and combined with other qualifications. Chemistry or Biology. General Studies excluded.	Acceptable combined with other qualifications. Biology at grade B and Chemistry at grade B required. General Studies excluded.	UKCAT compulsory Graduate entry available
Birmingham	AAB	Acceptable on its own and combined with other qualifications. Chemistry and either Biology or Physics or Mathematics. Human Biology may be offered, but not in addition to Biology. General Studies excluded.	Acceptable only when combined with other qualifications. Biology at AS level is required if not offered at A level. Human Biology may be offered instead of Biology.	Graduate entry available
Brighton and Sussex	340 tariff points	Acceptable on its own and combined with other qualifications. Biology or Chemistry required. General Studies excluded.	Acceptable combined with other qualifications. Chemistry and Biology. General Studies excluded.	UKCAT compulsory
Bristol	AAB	Acceptable on its own and combined with other qualifications. Chemistry at grade A required. General Studies excluded.	Acceptable combined with other qualifications. If four AS levels offered at least one should be in a non-science subject.	Graduate entry and Pre-Medical course available
Cambridge	AAA	Acceptable on its own and combined with other qualifications. One from	Acceptable only when combined with other qualifications. Three	BMAT compulsory

		Biology, Chemistry, Physics or Mathematics. Chemistry required at least to AS level.	of Biology, Chemistry, Physics, Mathematics.	Graduate entry available
Cardiff	370 tariff points	Acceptable on its own and combined with other qualifications. Two of Chemistry, Biology, Physics, Mathematics, Statistics.	Acceptable only when combined with other qualifications. Chemistry or Biology if not taken at A Level at grade B. General Studies excluded.	UKCAT compulsory Pre-Medical course available
Dundee	AAA	Acceptable on its own and combined with other qualifications. Chemistry and any science subject at grade A. General Studies excluded.	Not acceptable.	UKCAT compulsory Pre-Medical course available
East Anglia	AAB	Acceptable on its own and combined with other qualifications. Biology should be at least at B grade. General Studies excluded.	Acceptable only when combined with other qualifications.	UKCAT compulsory
Edinburgh	AAAb	Acceptable on its own and combined with other qualifications. Chemistry and any of Mathematics, Physics or Biology.	Acceptable only when combined with other qualifications. Biology required if not held at A level.	UKCAT compulsory Pre-Medical course available
Glasgow	AAB	Acceptable on its own and combined with other qualifications. Chemistry required and one from Biology, Mathematics or Physics. Biology or Human Biology in addition to Chemistry is preferred.	Acceptable only when combined with other qualifications.	UKCAT compulsory
Guy's, King's and St Thomas',	AABc	Acceptable on its own and combined with other qualifications. Biology at	Acceptable only when combined with other qualifications.	UKCAT compulsory Graduate entry

(cont.)

Table 3.1. For applicants with qualifications from England, Wales and Northern Ireland (*cont.*)

University	Grade			
London		grade B or Chemistry at grade B required. General Studies excluded.	General Studies excluded.	and Pre-Medical course available
Hull York	AABb	Acceptable on its own and combined with other qualifications. Chemistry and Biology required. General Studies excluded.	Acceptable only when combined with other qualifications. Biology and Chemistry required.	UKCAT compulsory
Imperial College, London	AABb	Acceptable on its own and combined with other qualifications. Biology or Chemistry required. General Studies excluded.	Acceptable combined with other qualifications. Biology and Chemistry required. General Studies excluded.	BMAT compulsory
Keele	AAB	Grades AAB required from Chemistry plus either Biology/Physics/Maths plus one further academic subject if only two sciences are offered.	Not acceptable.	UKCAT compulsory
Leeds	AAB	Acceptable on its own and combined with other qualifications. Chemistry required. General Studies excluded.	Acceptable only when combined with other qualifications.	UKCAT compulsory
Leicester	AAB	Acceptable on its own and combined with other qualifications. Chemistry required at grade A. General Studies excluded.	Acceptable combined with other qualifications. Biology and Chemistry required. General Studies excluded.	UKCAT compulsory; Graduate entry available
Liverpool	AAB	Acceptable on its own and combined with other qualifications. Chemistry required at grade A.	Acceptable combined with other qualifications. Biology and Chemistry required. General Studies acceptable.	Graduate entry available
Manchester	AAB	Acceptable on its own and combined with other qualifications. Chemistry and one other of Biology, Physics, Human Biology or Mathematics. General Studies excluded.	Acceptable only when combined with other qualifications. General Studies excluded.	UKCAT compulsory; Pre-Medical course available

University	Grades		
Newcastle	AAA	Acceptable on its own and combined with other qualifications. Chemistry or Biology required. General Studies excluded.	Acceptable only when combined with other qualifications.	UKCAT compulsory Graduate entry available
Nottingham	AAB	Acceptable on its own and combined with other qualifications. Chemistry and Biology (or Human Biology) at A grade. General Studies excluded.	Acceptable only when combined with other qualifications.	UKCAT compulsory Graduate entry available
Oxford	AAA	Acceptable on its own and combined with other qualifications. Chemistry with either Mathematics or Biology or Physics.	Acceptable only when combined with other qualifications. General Studies excluded.	UKCAT compulsory for graduate entry BMAT compulsory for undergraduate entry Graduate entry available
Peninsula	370 tariff points	Acceptable on its own and combined with other qualifications. Biology or Chemistry or Mathematics or Physics plus two further subjects at A level, preferably to include one non-science subject.	Acceptable combined with other qualifications. General Studies excluded.	UKCAT compulsory
Queens University, Belfast	AAAa	Acceptable only when combined with other qualifications. Chemistry at grade A and (Biology at grade A or Mathematics at grade A or Physics at grade A). General Studies excluded.	Acceptable only when combined with other qualifications. General Studies excluded.	
Sheffield	AAB	Acceptable on its own and combined with other qualifications. Chemistry and any Science subject.	Acceptable only when combined with other qualifications. Chemistry, Biology and one other science subject recommended.	UKCAT compulsory Pre-Medical course available

(cont.)

Table 3.1. For applicants with qualifications from England, Wales and Northern Ireland (*cont.*)

Southampton	AAB	Acceptable on its own and combined with other qualifications. Chemistry required.	Acceptable only when combined with other qualifications.	UKCAT compulsory Graduate entry available
St Andrews	AAB	Acceptable on its own and combined with other qualifications. Chemistry and Biology, Mathematics or Physics. General Studies excluded.	Acceptable only when combined with other qualifications.	UKCAT compulsory
St George's, London	AABb–BBCb	Acceptable on its own and combined with other qualifications. Chemistry and Biology required. General Studies excluded.	Not acceptable.	UKCAT compulsory Graduate entry available
Swansea	Graduate entry course.	Partnership arrangement with Cardiff for five-year medical degree. Contact medical school for further details.		Graduate entry available
University College London	AABe	Acceptable on its own and combined with other qualifications. Chemistry Biology required.	Acceptable only when combined with other qualifications.	BMAT compulsory
Warwick	Graduate entry course.	Candidates are expected to have a first class or good upper second class degree in Biological Sciences. Relevant work experience is essential.		Graduate entry available

Table 3.2. For applicants with qualifications from Scotland

University	Higher grades required	Subjects	Advanced Higher grades required	Subjects
Aberdeen	AAAAB	Three from Chemistry, Biology, Maths and Physics. Chemistry is desirable, only acceptable in one sitting.	ABB	Three from Chemistry, Biology, Maths and Physics. Chemistry is desirable, only acceptable in one sitting.
Barts, London, Queen Mary's	AAA	Acceptable only when combined with other qualifications. Chemistry and Biology required.	BB	Acceptable on its own and combined with other qualifications. Biology or Chemistry required.
Birmingham	AAAAB	Acceptable when combined with other qualifications. Two Advanced Higher also required.	–	Acceptable only when combined with other subjects.
Brighton and Sussex	340 tariff points	Biology and Chemistry. At least two Advanced Highers are also required. If you have studied Biology or Chemistry to Higher level only, you will additionally be expected to pass this subject at grade B.	–	Biology or Chemistry. Acceptable on its own and combined with other qualifications. At least two advanced highers required.
Bristol	AAAAA	Acceptable only when combined with other qualifications. Chemistry required.	AB	Acceptable only when combined with other qualifications. Chemistry required.
Cambridge	–	Acceptable only when combined with other qualifications.	AAA–AAB	Acceptable on its own and combined with other qualifications. One from Biology, Chemistry, Mathematics or Physics. Chemistry required at least to Higher level.

(cont.)

Table 3.2. For applicants with qualifications from Scotland (*cont.*)

Cardiff	AAAAB	English and Biology and Chemistry and Physics required.	AA	Chemistry required.
Dundee	AAABB	Acceptable on its own and combined with other qualifications. Chemistry and any science subject.	Not acceptable. Entry based on first sitting of Highers, not Advanced Highers.	
East Anglia		Acceptable only when combined with other qualifications. Acceptable with two advanced highers.	AAB	Acceptable on its own and combined with other qualifications. Biology required at grade B.
Edinburgh	AAAAB	Chemistry and two from Biology, Mathematics and Physics.	–	Refer to medical school prospectus.
Glasgow	AAAAB	Chemistry and two from Mathematics, Physics and Biology or Human Biology. Acceptable on its own and combined with other qualifications.	–	
Hull York	AAAAB	Chemistry and Biology required, only acceptable in one sitting.	AB	Chemistry and Biology required.
Imperial	–	Acceptable only when combined with other qualifications. Acceptable when combined with Advanced Highers.	AAB	Acceptable on its own and combined with other qualifications. Biology and Chemistry required.
Keele	–	4–5 subjects at standard grade are required with good range of grades, including English Language and	AAB	Chemistry essential, plus one from Biology/Physics/Maths, plus one further academic

University				
				subject if only 2 sciences offered. Alternatively 2 Advanced Highers plus one new Higher at AAA may be offered.
Guy's, King's and St Thomas', London	BBC	Mathematics. Any science subject not offered at Advanced Higher/Higher level required at standard grade level instead.	AA	Acceptable on its own and combined with other qualifications. Chemistry and Biology required.
Leeds	AAAAB	Acceptable only when combined with other qualifications. Chemistry or Biology required.	BB	Individual cases considered.
Leicester	AAAAA	Individual cases considered.	AAB	Acceptable on its own and combined with other qualifications. Chemistry and Biology.
Liverpool	AAAAA–AAABB	Acceptable on its own and combined with other qualifications. Chemistry and Biology.	AA	Acceptable on its own and combined with other qualifications.Chemistry and Biology both at A grade.
Manchester	–	Acceptable only when combined with other qualifications.	AAB	Acceptable only when combined with other qualifications.
Newcastle	AAAAA	Chemistry and/or Biology at grade A and Mathematics.	–	Acceptable only when combined with other qualifications.
Nottingham	–		AAB	Acceptable on its own and combined with other qualifications.Chemistry and Biology at grade A.
Oxford	AAAAA–AAAAB	Acceptable only when combined with other qualifications.	AAA	Acceptable on its own and combined with other qualifications. Chemistry and one from Mathematics, Biology or Physics.

(cont.)

Table 3.2. For applicants with qualifications from Scotland (*cont.*)

Peninsula	370 tariff points	Acceptable only when combined with other qualifications. At least one Science and preferably one non-Science required. Only acceptable in one sitting.	–	Acceptable only when combined with other qualifications. At least one Science and preferably one non-Science required. Only acceptable in one sitting.
Queens University, Belfast	AAAAA	Acceptable on its own and combined with other qualifications. Chemistry at grade A and Biology at grade A.	AAA	Acceptable on its own and combined with other qualifications. Chemistry at grade A and (Biology at grade A and Mathematics at grade A or Physics at grade A).
Sheffield	AAAAB	Acceptable only when combined with other qualifications. Only acceptable in one sitting.	AB	Chemistry at grade A and Any Science subject at grade B. Only acceptable in one sitting.
Southampton	AAAAB	Chemistry required.	AB	Chemistry required.
St Andrew's	AAABB	Chemistry and at least one other from Physics, Biology or Mathematics.	–	Acceptable on its own and combined with other qualifications.
St George's, London	AAAAA–BBBBB	Acceptable only when combined with other qualifications. Biology and Chemistry required.	AAA–AAB	Acceptable only when combined with other qualifications. Biology and Chemistry required.
Swansea	Graduate entry course.	Partnership arrangement with Cardiff for five-year medical degree. Contact medical school for further details.	–	

University College London	–	Not acceptable.	AAB	–	Acceptable on its own and combined with other qualifications Chemistry and Biology required.
Warwick	Graduate entry course.	Candidates are expected to have a first class or good upper second class degree in Biological Sciences. Relevant work experience is essential.			

Notes

1. Always confirm requirements with medical school before applying (see Appendix 5).
2. Some medical schools use the UCAS tariff point system to designate entry requirements. A copy of the UCAS tariff guide can be downloaded at www.ucas.com/candq/tariff/tariff06.doc.
3. GCE entry requirements written as, for example, AABc, ask that the applicant has, in this instance, two A levels at grade A, one at grade B, and an AS level at grade C (designated by the lower case letter).
4. UKCAT = UK Clinical Aptitude Test.
5. BMAT = BioMedical Admissions Test (BMAT).

in the first 2 years of the medical course is more common in those who did not take biology at A level. All universities require good grades in science and mathematics at GCSE level if not offered at A level, together with English language.

The relative popularity with applicants of mathematics over biology does not indicate changed perception of the value of mathematics for medicine but reflects the general usefulness of mathematics for entry to alternative science courses. It may also be because good mathematicians (or average mathematicians with good teachers) can expect higher grades in mathematics than in the more descriptive subject of biology. A few applicants gain excellent grades at A level in four subjects; for example, chemistry, physics, biology, and mathematics or the less appropriate combination for medicine of chemistry, physics or biology, mathematics, and higher mathematics. It is a better strategy for admission to achieve three good grades than four indifferent ones.

Scottish Highers and Advanced Highers are the usual entry qualification offered by Scottish applicants, most of whom apply to study at Scottish medical schools. Scottish qualifications are accepted by medical schools in England, Wales, and Northern Ireland. The Scottish academic tests are accompanied by formal testing of core study skills needed for understanding a university course: personal effectiveness and problem-solving, communication, numeracy, and information technology.

Both the International Baccalaureate and the European Baccalaureate are acceptable entry qualifications at UK medical schools and rapidly increasing numbers of applicants offer those qualifications. Requirements vary at different schools and can be found in the UCAS publication. A few students enter medicine with BTEC/SCOT BTEC National Diploma Certificate. The Advanced General National Vocational Qualification (GNVQ) or General Scottish Vocational Qualification (GSVQ) are not generally accepted unless combined with other qualifications, although some universities are prepared to consider it on an individual basis. It is likely that a distinction would be required, along with a high grade in GCE A level, probably in chemistry.

For applicants who want to pursue a career in medicine but lack a science background, a solution lies in the form of a premedical/foundation course. These are 1-year long and provide students with good grades in non-science subjects the opportunity to study basic science, providing a route into studying the full medical degree. Medical schools that currently offer foundation courses are Bristol, Cardiff, Dundee, Edinburgh, Guy's King's & St Thomas' London, Manchester, and Sheffield (see Table 3.1).

Alternatively, many medical schools in the UK will accept as an entry qualification the Access to Medicine Certificate from the College of West Anglia in King's Lynn (www.col-westanglia.ac.uk) and some also accept other access certificates. These are given for satisfactory completion of a 1-year full-time course in physics, chemistry, and biology designed for potential applicants to medical schools with good academic backgrounds or professional qualifications, such as in nursing (see Appendix 6).

It is clear from the complexity of the entry requirements discussed that no single process for selection exists at UK medical schools. Only with the recent advent of UKCAT has the standardisation of medical admissions been enhanced. The UK Clinical Aptitude Test (UKCAT) is currently used in the selection process by 23 of the 30 UK university Medical and Dental Schools: more than 20,000 would-be medical students sat the UKCAT between July and October of 2006. By focusing on the cognitive powers and attributes deemed valuable to health care professionals (rather than on specific curriculum or science content) the test seeks to select candidates whose mental abilities, attitudes, and professional behaviours are most appropriate for a clinical career but it would be fair to say that validation of the test is difficult. Nevertheless, the test probably helps universities to make more informed choices from amongst the many highly qualified applicants who apply for their medical and dental degree programmes.

If you are applying to a medical school that now requires the UKCAT, you should ideally take the test before applying to the medical school through UCAS. If you have any doubt about whether you are required to take the UKCAT, you should contact the universities to which you are planning to apply. Further information, including the list of medical schools requiring this test can be found on the UKCAT website www.ukcat.ac.uk.

The BioMedical Admissions Test (BMAT) is similar to the UKCAT in that it is a subject-specific admissions test taken by applicants to certain medicine and veterinary medicine courses. It is however less widely available than UKCAT and has similar validation problems. Further information can be found at www.bmat.org.uk.

Graduate students

Most medical schools will accept applications from graduates for the conventional course. A first- or upper second-class honours degree is usually required, most commonly in a science or health-related subject. Unless their degree includes chemistry or biochemistry, an A level in chemistry is usually required in addition. It may be acceptable for a graduate to sit the GAMSAT (Graduate Australian Medical School Admissions Test), a scientific aptitude test which is usually held once a year, for example at St George's Hospital Medical School. A good score in this, in addition to their degree and personal characteristics, may be acceptable. Students wishing to pursue this method of entry are best advised to contact their preferred schools early to discuss this option. In addition several medical schools have started fast-track (4 year) medical courses for some graduates (see Table 4.3). These courses generally condense the early years and basic science component of the course. Similarly those schools with 6-year courses that include an intercalated BSc or equivalent, such as Oxford, Imperial College, and Royal Free and University College Medical School, are introducing shorter (5 year) courses if you already have a similar degree. If the degree includes chemistry or biochemistry, it may be accepted in lieu of A level chemistry, otherwise this is likely to be required in addition. Graduate entrants are not normally exempted from any parts of the medical course at most medical schools but they are in some.

How about resits?

What about those who take longer before a first attempt or retake examinations after further study, having failed to achieve their grade target at first attempt? Clearly, there are perfectly understandable reasons for poor performance at first attempt, such as illness, bereavement, and multiple change of school, which most medical schools are prepared to take into account, at least if they had judged the candidate worthy of an offer in the first place. Medical schools which did not give an offer first time round are unlikely to make an offer at second attempt. Apart from these exceptions, most medical schools are not normally prepared to consider applicants who failed to obtain high grades at first attempt.

Three points might be made about applicants who, for no good reason, perform below target at first attempt. Firstly, a modest polishing of grades confers little additional useful knowledge and gives no promise of improved potential for further development, especially when only one or two subjects are retaken. The less there is to do the better it should be done, and the medical course itself requires the ability to keep several subjects on the boil simultaneously. On the other hand, a dramatic improvement (unless achieved by highly professional cramming) may indicate late development or reveal desirable and necessary qualities of determination and application. Secondly, age should be taken into account. The usual age for taking A level is 18 years, and some much younger applicants may simply have been taken through school too fast. Thirdly, those unlikely to achieve ABB at GCE A level (or equivalent) at first attempt are probably unwise to be thinking of medicine, unless their non-academic credentials are very strong indeed. Even then, it is likely to be an uphill battle. Read the prospectus carefully between the lines to try to discover those medical schools most likely to give weight to broader achievements.

Survival ability

So much for what we think medical schools are, or should be, looking for. But what qualities are needed for survival? We asked Susan Spindler, Producer of *Doctors to Be*, what in her opinion, based on several years in medical school and hospital making the television series, makes a good medical student. This is what she said:

Medical school is very hard work and great fun. There will be a vast array of things to do in your free time coupled with a syllabus that could have you working day and night for years. You need to be the sort of person who can keep both opportunities and work requirements in perspective. There is a lot of drinking and a lot of sport. In many universities the burden of the curriculum and the emotional pressure of the course means that medics tend to stick together and intense, but rather narrow, friendships can result. Try to make and maintain friendships with non-medics. Many medical schools aim to select gregarious, confident characters who have experience of facing and overcoming challenges and leading others. It certainly helps if you fit this mould – but there are many successful exceptions. You'll get the most out of medical school if you are impelled by some sort of desire to help others and blessed with boundless curiosity. You'll need the maturity and memory to handle a large volume of sometimes tedious learning; the ability to get on with people from all walks of life and a genuine interest in them; and sufficient humility to cope cheerfully with being at the bottom of the medical hierarchy for five years. It helps if you are good at forging strong and sustaining friendships – you'll need them when times get hard – and if you have some sort of moral and ethical value system that enables you to cope with the accelerated experience of life's extremes (birth, death, pain, suicide, suffering) that you will get during medical school.

REMEMBER

- Academic ability is not the only quality needed to secure a place at medical school.

- Broader attributes, such as compassion, endurance, determination, communication skills, enthusiasm, intellectual curiosity, balance, adaptability, integrity, and a sense of humour are also needed.

- There are national guidelines regarding health and personal requirements to which all applicants must adhere. Failure to disclose information which may put patients at risk will result in losing a place at medical school.

- UK universities require AAB or higher at A level at first attempt, but this alone does not guarantee admission.

- A level chemistry (or physical science) is normally required but practically all of the medical schools will accept AS chemistry in its place. Biology is becoming the next preferred subject. All medical schools will accept at least one non-science A level.

- Scottish Advanced Highers and European/International Baccalaureate examinations are accepted at UK universities.

- Entry requirements for graduate applicants are more flexible, and options exist for some graduates to apply for shortened courses in some schools.

- Applicants who are resitting A levels will usually only be considered in special circumstances and should expect to be given higher entry requirements.

4

Choosing a medical school

The attitude that "beggars can't be choosers" is not only pessimistic but wrong. If, after serious consideration, you have decided that medicine is the right career for you and you are the right person for medicine, then the next step is to find a place at which to study where you can be happy and successful. This chapter is designed to help guide you into choosing the right schools to consider flirting with, rather than necessarily ending up (metaphorically speaking, of course) in bed with.

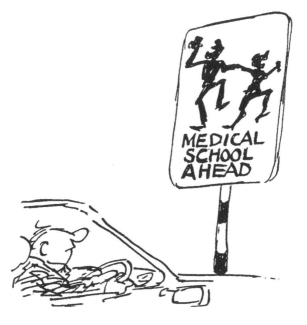

Walk into any medical school in the country and ask a bunch of the students which is the best medical school in the country and you will receive an almost universal shout of "This one, of course!" The general public's typical image of medical students is one of a group of young people who live life to the full, work hard, and play harder; hotheaded youngsters who can be excused their puerile pranks and mischievous misdemeanours, because, "Well, they must have a release from all that pressure, mustn't they". While this image should be treated with the same caution that is required with any stereotype, it nonetheless contains grains of truth. When you further consider the outstanding abilities of many medical students in their chosen extracurricular interests, it will come as no surprise to find that medical schools are full of students letting their hair down, getting involved in the things they enjoy, having a good time, and still doing enough work to pass those dreaded examinations and assessments, or at least most of the time anyway. The only dilemma you have is to find which of these centres of social excitement and intellectual challenge best suits your particular interests and nature. Like all the best decisions in life the only way to find out is to do a bit of groundwork and research, plan out the lay of the land, then follow your instincts and go for it.

Medical schools vary greatly in the size of their yearly intake (Table 4.1). It is difficult to offer more precise advice about discovering the "spirit" or "identity" of an institution. However hard it may be to define, all the medical schools possess a uniqueness of which they are rightly proud. Of course some schools wear their hearts more on their sleeves than others or have a more easily identifiable image, but often the traditional identities are past memories, especially in London, where medical schools' identities have changed considerably in the past decade, particularly with recent amalgamations between medical schools and their mergers with larger multidisciplinary university colleges.

In days gone by a choice had to be made between a hospital-based medical school, such as several in London, or an initially firmly multifaculty university environment, with a much broader student community with greater diversity of personalities, outlooks, and opportunities. This distinction has largely now disappeared; only the course at St George's in London is hospital and medical school based throughout.

Accommodation may play an important part in choice, as some colleges house all the medics in one hall of residence while others spread them out,

Table 4.1. Predicted size of entry to first year of standard course in medicine in UK medical schools for 2007

Over 350	Birmingham
	King's (University of London)
	Manchester
	Newcastle
Over 300	Cambridge
	Imperial (University of London)
	Leeds
	Liverpool
	Queen Mary's (University of London)
	UCL (University of London)
Over 200	Bristol
	Edinburgh
	Glasgow
	Nottingham
	Sheffield
	St George's, University of London
	UWCM, Cardiff
150–200	Aberdeen
	Dundee
	Leicester
	Oxford
	Peninsula
	Southampton
	Queen's, Belfast
	Warwick
Less than 150	Brighton-Sussex
	East Anglia
	Hull-York
	Keele
	St Andrew's
	Swansea

so you may end up living on a corridor with a lawyer, a historian, a musician, a dentist, a physicist, and someone who seems to sleep all day and smoke funny smelling tobacco who is allegedly doing "Media Studies and Ancient

Icelandic". Many find this kind of variety gives them exactly what they came to university for and would find spending all their work and play time with people on the same course socially stifling. While it is essentially a matter of personal preference, it is also worth noting that both have pros and cons; for example, when the workload is heavy it may be easier to knuckle down if everyone around you is doing likewise. Conversely, when a bunch of medics get together they inevitably talk medicine, and, although recounting tales and anecdotes can amuse many a dinner party it may well breed narrow individuals with a social circle limited only to other medics. Choosing a campus site or a city site where you live side by side with the community your hospital serves may also have a different appeal.

Increasing diversity is being introduced to the design of the curriculum and how it is delivered. The traditional method of spending 2 or 3 years studying the basic sciences in the isolation of the medical school and never seeing a patient until you embarked on the clinical part of the course has all but disappeared. The teaching of subjects is generally much more integrated both between the different departments and between clinical and preclinical aspects. Even so, some curricula are predominantly "systems based" and others "clinical problem based". Much more emphasis is being placed in all courses on clinical relevance, self-directed learning, and problem-solving rather than memorising facts given in didactic lectures. There is substantial variation in the extent to which these changes have evolved and in many respects there is greater choice between courses than ever before. Diversity of approach is a strength of the UK system: "You pay your money and take your choice".

The courses at Oxford, Cambridge, and St Andrews remain more traditional in structure if not in subject matter and teaching methods. These courses maintain a distinct separation between the more scientific and the more clinical, although they have moved away to some extent from separate subjects towards systems-based teaching of the sciences and have introduced reference to clinical relevance; their philosophy is that it is still valid to study in depth the sciences related to medicine (anatomy, physiology, biochemistry, pharmacology, and pathology) as disciplines important in their own right, primarily as tools of intellectual development and scientific education rather than of vocational equipment. Cambridge and Oxford, however, have also introduced a 4-year course for graduate students, which combines the intellectual rigour of the traditional course with community-based clinical insights from the outset.

At Oxford all the basic sciences required for the professional qualifications are covered in the intensive first five terms'work and are then examined in the first BM. All students then take in their remaining four terms the honours school in physiology, a course much wider than its name suggests with options to choose from all the basic medical sciences, including pathology and psychology.

Cambridge adopts a more flexible approach. All the essential components of the medical sciences course are covered in 2 years. The third year is spent either studying in depth one of a number of medically related subjects, or reading for a part II in any subject – law, music, or whatever takes their fancy – provided they have a suitable educational background and their local education authority is sufficiently inspired to support them. The 3 years lead to an honours BA.

At St Andrews the students spend 3 years studying for an ordinary degree or 4 years for an honours degree in medical sciences. Although strongly science based, clinical relevance is emphasised and some clinical insights are given, mainly in a community setting. Most St Andrews graduates go on to clinical studies at Manchester University, but a few go to other universities. By the year 2009 it is hoped that Scottish funding will enable St Andrews graduates to stay in Scotland – in Glasgow, Edinburgh, Aberdeen, and Dundee – for their clinical studies. The four 'newest' UK undergraduate medical schools include Peninsula Medical School (Universities of Exeter and Plymouth), University of East Anglia Medical School, Hull-York Medical School and Brighton and Sussex Medical School – these opened their doors to medical students in 2002 and 2003.

This then brings us back to those important but less tangible attractions of each medical school, the spirit and identity of the place. Unless you are an aficionado of architecture and simply could not concentrate unless in a neo-classical style lecture theatre or an art deco dissecting room, then what gives a place its unique character are the people who inhabit it; the biomedical science teachers, the hospital consultants who involve themselves in student life, the mad old dear who runs the canteen, the porter who knows everyone's name and most people's business, the all important dean and admissions tutor, and not least by any means the students themselves. It is the ever-changing student body that above all else shapes the identity of a school and certainly gives it spirit and expresses its ever-changing nature in a dynamic spirit. Just listen to any final-year student bemoaning how the old

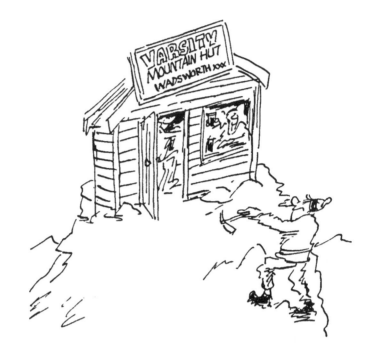

place has changed and how the new first year just are not the same as the rest of us and how what used to be like a rugby academy is more like a ballet school these days. What these oldies do not realise is that exactly the same was said 5 years ago when they were the freshers and 5 years before that and so on.

The most obvious expression of this spirit is the plethora of clubs and societies that grow up in every medical school. Whatever your fancy it is worth investigating what facilities could be on offer. There is little point in being determined to gain entry to a medical school to pursue your hobby in climbing mountains if there is no tradition of such activities at that college, especially when another equally good college in other respects has a climbing wall on campus, a mountaineering hut in the Lake District, and an alpine club which goes on annual trips to Switzerland.

Location

Most individuals will have some idea of what sort of medical school they are looking for. The first criterion is usually a suitable geographical location. Some prefer to stay nearer home, some cannot move away fast enough. Some want to be up north or down south, out in the sticks or right in the smoke. Almost all medical schools are in large cities within the academic centres of research and teaching, and where patients of endless variety are concentrated. Most medical schools, however, are making increasing use of associated district hospitals and primary care centres, such as general practice surgeries, in surrounding suburban and rural areas. This allows for a broader and more balanced experience and exposure to different medical conditions and practices.

If you wish to stay near home it is worth remembering that medical school accommodation may be limited, and consequently you may be given low priority and find yourself having to live at home. The downside is that those not living in halls of residence with their new friends and having to commute to and from home find it more difficult to immerse themselves in student life and may end up feeling isolated and unfulfilled by university life.

Finances

An increasingly important issue related to accommodation and other living costs which has to be considered is student debt. Surveys over the past 10 years have shown a consistent and alarming rise in the levels of debt for all students, in both the government student loans scheme and in overdrafts and loans from banks. The situation is worse for medical students because of the length of the course, the shorter vacations in the later years, and the intensive nature of the training and examinations limiting opportunities for part-time casual work. Other factors such as expensive books and equipment, and the need to dress appropriately also add to the cost; turning up to the professor's clinic attired in smelly old trainers, ragged jeans, and a Glastonbury T-shirt is hardly portraying a professional image.

The one advantage that medical students do have over many other students is that when they qualify they are pretty certain of falling into secure and reasonably well-paid jobs. Still, seeing a large chunk of your hard-earned first pay cheque disappear into the repayments of your several thousand pound debt is not a pleasant feeling, especially when the shackles of debt can last for several years after you leave medical school. The size of individuals' debts at the end of their time at medical school can vary enormously, depending on personal circumstances, but it is now not uncommon for final-year students to owe over £20,000, and in many cases considerably more: indeed, a BMA survey has revealed that the average medical student now owes more in debt than they will earn in their first year as a junior doctor.

The introduction of tuition fees of up to £3000 from 2006–2007 onwards is likely to worsen student debt – indeed it has already been blamed for a recent slump in medical school applications. These fees, better known as 'top-up' fees are the ones that attracted so much controversy a couple of years ago. They basically represent a new way of charging tuition to undergraduate students who study at universities in England and Wales. They are dependent upon where the student comes from and where they go to university so that English and Northern Irish students will pay top-up fees wherever they study in the UK, Welsh students will pay top-up fees in England, Scotland or Northern Ireland, but only the current £1250 a year fee if they remain in Wales or study a course elsewhere that is not available at any Welsh university, Scottish students will pay top-up fees in England, Wales or Northern Ireland; if they remain in Scotland, they will pay a £2145 endowment upon graduation (as is the case now), EU students will pay fees as if they came from the nation they are studying in (in other words, always the lowest amount), and International students will continue to pay their university's international fees, which are typically even higher than top-up fees.

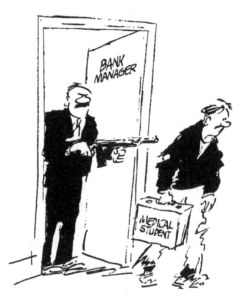

For overseas students who do not qualify for student loans and who have to pay full tuition fees, most schools expect proof of the ability not only to pay the fees but also of resources to live on during their time at medical school.

For mature students, particularly graduates, who may not qualify for the usual support from their local council, the Departments of Health for England and Wales now have a bursary scheme to support the last 3 years of training. The amounts which will be paid vary according to the student's individual case, for instance if they have children to support or other income sources. More information can be obtained by reading *Financial Help for Healthcare Students* (Seventh edition) (which is available online at www.doh.gov.uk/hcsmain.htm) or by contacting National Health Service (NHS) Careers (Tel: 0845 6060655).

It would be sensible then to consider that in choosing your medical school some areas are obviously more expensive to live in than others. It should not, however, completely put you off these areas because many students in London or Edinburgh, for instance, believe that the advantages they have of being in such a place are well worth the extra expense. It is therefore worth finding out about the cost and availability of accommodation and general living expenses at any school that you are keen on.

Range of entrance requirements

Choice of medical school must be guided by a realistic expectation of the chances of achieving its basic entrance requirements. This does not just mean will you reach the right grades, all of which are between ABB and AAA for A levels but, more importantly, have you done acceptable subjects, and acceptable examinations (see p. 33).

Overseas students from outside the European Union (EU) should check with medical authorities in their own country which medical schools will provide them with a qualification that will be recognised at home, as not all UK medical degrees may be acceptable. Overseas students should check the quota allowed for each school and whether any particular criteria are used in selecting applicants; for example, if priority is given to students from the developing world or countries with historic links to one school or another or to students without a medical school in their own country.

A gap year?

Most schools now encourage students to take a gap year if they want to, although it is not a requirement. It is important, however, to follow some basic ground rules. Firstly, if you are planning a gap year, ensure you mark your UCAS form for deferred entry. Although you can apply for this retrospectively, it is much more likely that schools will agree to your request if they know about it as early as possible. Secondly, have some firm plans of what you want to do in your year out and why. It is something you should write, albeit briefly, in your personal statement and is a common topic for questioning in an interview. Your year out does not need to be spent doing anything medical, but you may want it to be, nor does it always have to involve travelling to the four corners of the earth. Finally, it is worth remembering that 5 or 6 years at medical school for most people means a considerable financial debt. So if you can spend some time earning some money, it will certainly come in useful; whatever you do, do not start your course already burdened with a large overdraft and credit card bills. Most of all, enjoy your gap year; it will give you lots of experiences you will never forget and be a great preparation for life as a student.

Interview or no interview

If you have a fear of interviews or an objection to being selected on the basis of an interview then there are schools which still do not interview (Table 4.2), despite the trend towards more schools adopting the interview as a useful adjunct to the confidential reference, the academic record, and the student's own comments on the UCAS form. It is worth remembering that interviews vary in terms of length, panel composition, structure, content and scoring methods. The best advice is this: prepare to be greeted by a minimum of two examiners, know your personal statement and medical school prospectus inside out, and think before launching into answers.

Visits and open days

In summary, there are numerous factors which prospective students should take into consideration when deciding which medical schools to apply to,

Table 4.2. Interviewing policies of UK medical school according to whether or not they normally interview shortlisted applicants

Aberdeen	Yes
Birmingham	Yes
Brighton and Sussex	Yes
Bristol	Yes
Cambridge	Yes
Dundee	Yes
East Anglia	Yes
Edinburgh	No, only short-listed graduate and mature applicants
Glasgow	Yes
Hull-York	Yes
Imperial College, London	Yes
Keele	Yes
King's College, London	Yes
Leeds	Yes
Leicester-Warwick	Yes
Liverpool	Yes
Manchester	Yes
Newcastle	Yes
Nottingham	Yes
Oxford	Yes
Peninsula	Yes
Queen Mary's, London	Yes
Queen's University, Belfast	No
Sheffield	Yes
Southampton	No, only short-listed graduate/ mature/international applicants
St Andrews	No, only interview mature applicants and a proportion of school leavers
St George's, London	Yes
University College, London	Yes
University of Wales College of Medicine, Cardiff	Yes

some relevant to all students and some specific to special cases. The most important advice is to visit as many schools as possible, take in the general feel of the place, look at the accommodation and facilities, explore the local area, and especially take time to talk to the current students, most of whom will, of course, be biased in favour of their school but who will at least be able to enthuse about the good points and answer your questions. Open days and sixth form conferences provide a more formal opportunity to do this. Later, a visit for interview may reinforce first impressions. A particularly good opportunity to compare medical schools is provided by the Medlink conference held in Nottingham in December each year. Most medical schools are represented and you will have opportunity to ask questions informally (visit www.medlink-uk.com).

A little careful groundwork can not only improve your chances of obtaining a place at a medical school but also help you to ensure that that place is at the right school in which to spend some of the best years of your life.

Graduate entry medicine

One response to the Department of Health initiative to not only increase the number of doctors in the UK but also provide a different breed of doctors for the future (GMC "Tomorrow's Doctors") has been the surge in graduate entry programmes. To date, over 715 places exist in UK medical schools for graduates keen to change direction and embark on a career in medicine.

Certainly the direction change can be acute. Whether making the leap from an arts background, scaling another rung of the health-care career ladder, or returning to formal education from the office, each and every graduate is faced with four intensive years of medical training. Say goodbye to long summer holidays!

The perks? First of all, speed; as a mature student it is natural to be concerned that you are making a "late" decision, that you are just starting out whilst contemporaries of your first degree are settled in a cosy world of work. Concerns of this kind can to some extent be assuaged by the fact that "fast-track" courses do just that, covering the same amount in four years as a standard course does in five or six. Furthermore, this intensity of medical training (demanding though it is) confers another advantage; science and clinical medicine are learnt side by side from the word go. Theories are put into practice.Complex disease mechanisms are contextualised in a world beyond the textbook. The perks of the financial climate in which graduate medics find themselves are less overt. The current situation is that students pay maximum tuition fees only in year one. For this they are eligible for a maximum means-tested student loan. After that, students can apply for a Department of Health Bursary and a 50% means-tested student loan. So, whenever your mind is saddened by all the synonyms of "student life" – baked beans, plastic cup coffee, dread of the hole in the wall's "Now check your account?" proposal – be uplifted not only by the success stories of many a mature student doctor but also by that oft forgot wonder: the student card!

All graduate entry programmes are identical in their length of course (four years), their interviewing process (all shortlisted applicants are interviewed), and in the fact that their intake is currently restricted to home and EU students only (Table 4.3). Beyond that similarities end. Choosing the right course for you takes careful consideration. An informed decision will assess location, style of teaching (whether problem-based (PBL) or traditional learning), and length of establishment of medical school.

PBL was pioneered as a teaching method in the 1960s in Canada. Straying from the traditional rote learning it claims to promote lasting learning that is more readily applicable to relevant contexts. In terms of medical teaching, PBL involves small groups of medical students being given a clinical case that triggers both individual and communal investigation of the relevant basic science. Success depends on self direction, sharing of knowledge, and collaboration. For example, St George's is strictly PBL whilst Cambridge is more traditional. Others such as Newcastle combine both methods of learning.

With their first student intakes in 2003 and 2004, the most recent established fast-track courses include Bristol, King's, Liverpool, Nottingham, Southampton, and Swansea.

The main factor dictating choice of medical school will be the entry criteria each course sets. To apply for the fast-track medical degree candidates need a minimum of a 2:2 in their previous degree. The nature of that degree is relevant – do not waste an application on a course that cites "Life Science" if your first degree was in History of Art! Certainly, humanities graduates can, indeed are welcomed to study medicine. Currently, there are

Table 4.3. Graduate Entry Medicine courses for 2007 (including minimal entry requirements and number of places)

Medical school	Minimum entry requirements	Number of places
Barts and the London Queen Mary's	2:1 Honours in science discipline	45
Birmingham	2:1 Honours in science discipline, Chemistry grade C at A level	42
Bristol	2:1 Honours in science discipline	19
Cambridge	2:1 Honours in any discipline	20
Guy's, King's, and St Thomas's	2:1 Honours in any discipline or 2:2 plus Postgraduate Degree/ Diploma in Nursing with 2 years experience	27
Leicester	2:1 Honours in science discipline	61
Liverpool	2:1 Honours in science discipline	33
Newcastle	2:1 Honours in any discipline	25
Nottingham	2:2 Honours in any discipline	91
Oxford	2:1 Honours in science discipline and 2 science A levels	30
Southampton	2:1 Honours in any discipline, GCSE passes in English, Maths, Science, AS passes in Chemistry and Biology or A level pass in Chemistry	40
St George's	2:2 Honours in any discipline	71
Swansea	2:1 Honours in any discipline, GCSE English grade B and Maths grade C, post-GCSE experience in Biology/ Chemistry	42
Warwick	2:1 Honours in science discipline	169

seven fast-track courses that welcome applications from non-science graduates: Cambridge, King's, Newcastle, Nottingham, Southampton, St George's and Swansea. Peter McCrorie, pioneer of the fast-track course at St George's, explains the move to widen access to medical training,

Which graduates should we admit? Scientific knowledge is core to a medical degree, so science qualifications are usually demanded for entry to medicine. But what about those who chose arts and humanities at school and university but now want to change direction? Study of the humanities has been shown to correlate with better clinical performance, so ideally both scientific knowledge and ability in the humanities should contribute. The solution at St George's Hospital was to invite applicants with any degree subject and give them an exam that covers both science and the humanities. We adopted the Graduate Australian Medical School Admission Test (GAMSAT), a broad based exam that covers scientific knowledge and reasoning in the humanities and includes two short essays to assess ability to argue logically and communicate in writing.

Nottingham and Swansea also use GAMSAT as part of their selection process. It is worth researching this website (gamsat@ucas.co.uk) or calling the UCAS Gamsat Office on 01242 544730 for practice papers and application, and examination dates before launching on regardless.

MSAT is another admissions test offered by some medical schools as an alternative to GAMSAT. Instead of assessing reasoning in basic sciences directly it focuses on the general "extra-curricular" skills and personal attributes that complement academic achievement. It caters for students applying to both undergraduate and graduate entry programmes Where Cambridge, Kings, Newcastle, and Southampton cite A level chemistry as an entry requirement, a number of Access to Medicine Courses have sprung up to cater to this need. These generally last one academic year and equip you with the scientific basis necessary both for the GAMSAT and for year one of a medicine degree (see Appendix 6).

The relative novelty of these GEM courses in the UK (our first programme was set up at St George's in 2000) mean that performance assessments of fast-track doctors are somewhat problematic. If Australia and America are anything to go by, then we can only be encouraged by the results – graduate course doctors on the wards have been proven to fare as well, and sometimes even better, than undergraduate ones. Who knows, maybe Kevin Hayes, senior lecturer in obstetrics and gynaecology at St George's is right in his forecast of an entirely graduate entry system of medical education in the future: "It wouldn't surprise me if in 30 years' time there are no school leavers doing medicine".

Experience of an arts graduate on the first year of a fast-track course

Having studied English and Philosophy as my first degree, beginning the Cambridge Graduate Course in Medicine was like arriving in a foreign country where I didn't speak the language. Most of my course mates were accomplished scientists with matching vocabularies, and I had never felt so stupid. Once I got used to the idea that the only question I would be asking in supervisions was 'Could you repeat that again please, and more slowly', my head was above water. My course mates and supervisors served as excellent translators and by the end of the first term I was amazed by what I had learned. The advantage of having a more naïve background was that as science unravelled its secrets, I found I could be left genuinely gob-smacked. However it was my toughest year yet academically. My most reluctant adaptation was to the scientist's language-destroying penchant for acronyms.

In the "holidays" we went to hospital for clinical experience. Here everyone was on a more even footing, and the pace more humane. Getting hands on experience was fun and exciting, and patient contact made me realise the value of all the swotting and communication skills acquired in my former lives. Both doctors and patients were so encouraging and personally I enjoyed escaping the Cambridge bubble once in a while. It was tough at Easter when we were trying to revise for summer exams as well as get the most out of clinical attachments, but we were all in it together. A huge benefit of an intensive course was the camaraderie amongst such a diverse bunch of people.

The summer exams, having appeared like thunder-clouds on the horizon in Spring, were less terrifying close up. Many of us were pleased to have some unstructured time in which to study in a way that suited us. They were without doubt the hardest exams I have sat, but the pass marks were low, and miraculously I passed them all first time.

Regarding the horror stories about sacrificing your whole life to medicine: it is very demanding but not all consuming. Most people can have a social life, play sport, maintain a long-distance relationship or acquire a new one, as well as study medicine.

It has been a busy, stressful, fulfilling year that I would recommend to anyone. My major gripe is that I have learnt thousands of new words and I am still crap at Scrabble.

HAW

REMEMBER

- Medical schools vary greatly in size, location, and style.

- Most, but not all, medical schools are in large cities, but often use hospitals and health centres in nearby towns and villages for teaching attachments.

- Cost of living can vary considerably between different parts of the country.

- Availability and quality of accommodation and leisure facilities should be considered.

- Living at home costs less, but most students prefer to move away from home and widen their experience.

- Courses are all giving increasing emphasis to clinical relevance and experience in the early years, but some have more than others.

- Only one school, St George's, is entirely hospital campus based throughout.

- Check up on the medical school's attitude to overseas students and mature applicants if relevant to you.

- Many opportunities now exist for graduates to apply for shortened courses.

- Most importantly do your homework, read the prospectuses (most universities publish an official one and an "alternative prospectus" written by students), read the online prospectus or course outline and selection criteria on the school's web site, attend open days, careers fairs, Medlink conferences, or ring medical schools to arrange to look round; most will be happy to oblige, you can get a feel for the place, check out the facilities, and you will be able to ask questions of students already there.

5

Application and selection

The whole emphasis of this book is to aid and encourage potential medical students to examine properly the career they are considering. This chapter deals in more detail with some of the practical "nuts and bolts" of the process of applying to and being selected by a medical school. All too often careers advice concentrates too much on these practicalities, implying the only criteria for choosing future doctors are whether they can fill out an impressive application form and get themselves selected. This detracts from the more important process of your addressing medicine's suitability as a career for you, and your suitability to be a doctor. Only after giving this serious consideration should you consider the details of application and selection set out in this chapter.

Unfortunately, the qualities which count for most in medicine are not precisely measurable. The measurable – examination performance at school – neither necessarily relates to these qualities nor guarantees intellectual or practical potential. Stewart Wolfe, an American physician, was right to ask:

Are the clearly specified and hence readily defensible criteria those most likely to yield a wise and cultivated doctor – a person capable of dealing with uncertainty, of compassionate understanding and wise judgment? Can an ideal physician be expected from an intellectual *forme fuste* who has spent his college years only learning the "right answers"?

Furthermore, there is no acceptable objective measure of the quality of the doctor against which to test the validity of selection decisions. In this sea of uncertainty, it is not surprising that selection processes are open to criticism.

Nonetheless, few patients would choose a doctor without meeting him or her first and a strong argument can be made for discovering the people behind their Universities' and Colleges' Admissions Service (UCAS) forms, if only briefly. Also, many applicants think that they should have an opportunity to put their own case for becoming a doctor.

Selection for interview (and at some schools for offer without interview) is made on the strength of an application submitted through UCAS. An application is completed partly by the applicant (either online or on paper) and partly by a referee, usually the head or a member of the school staff, who submits a confidential reference.

Altogether, about 19,000 home and European Union (EU) and overseas applicants compete for about 8000 places to read medicine at universities. Women comprise over half (56%) of all applicants and entrants. In 2008, over 700 of the home and EU places will be on fast-track graduate courses.

It is worth completing the UCAS form accurately and legibly. Deans and admission tutors who have to scan a thousand or two application forms (which they receive reduced in size from the original application) simply do not have time to spend deciphering illegible handwriting. A legible, even stylish, presentation creates a good impression from the start.

Personal details

The first section of the UCAS form presents the personal details of the applicant, including age on 30 September of the coming academic year. Many applicants give their current age instead and at a glance seem to fall below the minimum age for entry at some medical schools or to be so young that older applicants might reasonably be given priority over them. True, the date of birth is also requested, but the quickly scanning eye may not pick up the discrepancy.

The list of schools attended by an applicant is often a useful guide to the educational opportunity received. More ability and determination are needed to emerge as a serious candidate for medicine from an unselective school with 2000 pupils, of whom only 10–15 normally enter university each year, than from a selective school for which university entry is the norm.

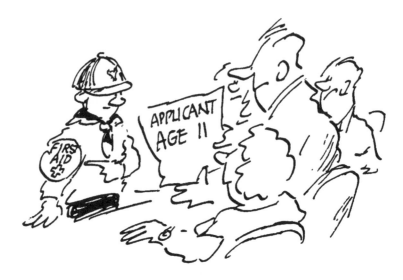

Choices

Applicants are not expected to give all their course choices to medicine. Six university courses can be nominated on UCAS forms, and the medical schools have requested that applicants should limit the number of applications for medicine to four. The remaining choices can be used for an alternative course without prejudice to the applications for medicine. You should remember, however, that if a backup offer for a non-medical course is accepted and the candidate fails to get the grades for medical school but does sufficiently well for the backup then that offer has to be accepted, and it is not possible to enter clearing for medicine. The only alternative is to withdraw from university entry in that year and to apply again the following year.

Other information

Examination results should be clearly listed by year. It is sensible to list first those subjects immediately relevant to the science requirements for medicine and then those subjects needed for university matriculation, usually English language and mathematics. All attempts at examinations should be entered and clearly separated. The date and number of A level or degree examinations yet to be taken complete the picture.

While it probably never pays to try to amuse on an application form, it is worth being interesting. Your personal statement presents an opportunity to catch the eye of a tired admissions dean because medicine demands so much more than academic ability, so include mention of your outside interests and experiences. John Todd, a consultant physician, observed from his own experience that:

The value of the physician is derived far more from what may be called his general qualities than from his special knowledge … such qualities as good judgment, the ability to see a patient as a whole, the ability to see all aspects of a problem in the right perspective and the ability to weigh up evidence are far more important than the detailed knowledge of some rare syndrome.

Small details, such as the information that an applicant spends his free moments delivering newspapers, assisting in the village shop, and acting as "pall bearer and coffin carrier to the local undertaker" converts a cipher into a person. None of those particular activities may be immediately relevant to future medical practice but at least they show initiative. Other activities, such as hobbies, music, drama, and sport, indicate a willingness and ability to acquire intellectual and practical skills and to participate, characteristics useful in life in general but also to a medical school which needs its own cultural life to divert tired minds and to develop full personalities during a long course of training.

Some applicants offer a remarkably wide variety of accomplishments, such as the boy who declared in his UCAS form: "I play various types of music, including jazz, Irish traditional, orchestral, and military band, on trombone, fiddle, tin whistle, mandolin, and bodhran. …" If Irish music be the food of medicine, play on. But that was not all, for he continued: "I also enjoy boxing and I have a brown belt (judo). My more social pastimes include ballroom dancing, photography, driving, and motor cycling". Would this young man have time for medicine?

It is not sensible to enter every peripheral interest and pastime lest it appears, as indeed may be so, that many of these activities are superficial. It is also unwise for an applicant to enter any interest that he or she would be unable to discuss intelligently at interview.

The applicant's own account of interests and the confidential report (for which a whole page is available) sometimes bring to life the different sides of an applicant's character. For example, one young man professed "a great interest in music" and confessed that he was "lead vocalist in a rowdy pop group" while his headmaster reported that he was "fairly quiet in lessons … science and medicine afford him good motivation … his choice of career suits him well. There is no doubt that he has the ability and temperament successfully to follow his calling". All in all this interplay of information is useful, for medicine is a suitable profession for multifaceted characters.

The confidential report is always important and is sometimes crucial. Most teachers take great care to give a balanced, realistic assessment of progress and potential in these confidential reports. Readers of UCAS forms quickly discover the few schools pupilled entirely by angels. Cautionary nuances are more commonly conveyed by what is omitted than by what is said, but a few heads are sufficiently outspoken to write from the hip in appropriate circumstances. Euphemisms may or may not be translated such as: "Economy of effort and calm optimism have been the hallmark of his academic process. Put another way, his teachers used to complain of idleness and lack of interest". Others indicate that they are attempting to get the candidate to come to terms with reality. For example: "We have explained to him that you are not in the business to supply fairy tale endings to touching UCAS references and that you will judge him on his merits".

It sounded as if that candidate was likely to come to the same fate as he would be an officer cadet rejected from Sandhurst with the explanation that "he sets himself extremely low standards – unfortunately he totally fails to live up to them". Not that every head gets it right, like the one whose pen slipped in writing: "Ian also has the distinction of being something of an expert in breeding erotic forms of rabbits".

Fair but frank confidential references are an essential part of an acceptable selection process. The confidential report usually includes a prediction of performance at A level, useful because it is set in the context of the report as a whole; but predictions can be misleading. A recent survey of the accuracy of A level predictions indicated that only about one third turned out to be correct, a half were too high (and half of these by two or more grades) and a tenth were too low. Occasionally a candidate is seriously underestimated, with the result that an interview is not offered and the applicant is at the mercy of the clearing procedure after the results are declared or has to apply again next year. Application to medical school after the results are known would be fairer but the practical difficulties in changing the system have so far proved insuperable.

Getting an interview

What in the mass of information counts most in the decision to shortlist a candidate for interview or even, at some medical schools, an offer without interview? Grades achieved in General Certificate of Secondary Education (GCSE) and A level if already taken or predicted grades if not yet taken are universally important. Medical schools also take notice of, but may give different weighting to, outstanding achievement in any field because excellence is not lightly achieved. They look for evidence of determination, perseverance, and consideration for others; for an ability to communicate; for breadth and depth of other interests, especially to signs of originality; for the contribution likely to be made to the life of the medical school; for a solid confidential report; and for assessment of potential for further development by taking all the evidence together. Highly though achievement is valued, potential, both personal and intellectual, is even more important. Perceptive shortlisters look for applicants who are just beginning to get into their stride in preference to those who have already been forced to their peak, aptly described by Dorothy L. Sayers in *Gaudy Night* as possessed of "small summery brains that flower early and run to seed". Although the shortlisting process deliberately sets out to view applicants widely, analysis of the outcome has shown that academic achievement still carries the weight in selecting candidates from their UCAS forms. The great majority of applicants called for interview are academically strong, and it is then that their personal characteristics decide the outcome (see Chapter 6).

What weight is put on medically related work experience in shortlisting – and what indeed is "medically related"? If you look through the stated views of individual medical schools in the *UCAS Guide to Entry to Medicine* on the "qualities" they are seeking in applicants, you will find three constantly recurring themes: communication skills, evidence of concern for the welfare of others, and a realistic perception of what medicine entails. It follows that any work experience that entails dealing with the public, actively helping or caring for others, or which shows doctors at work and health care in action may enable you to be convincing in establishing your ability to communicate,

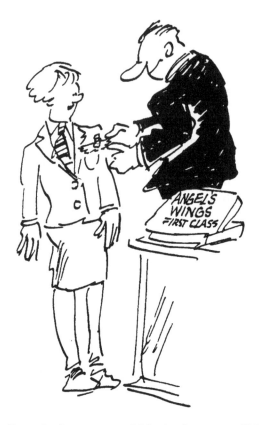

your understanding of what you would be letting yourself in for, and your discovery of the skills and attributes you already possess which makes you suitable in principle for the responsibilities of a doctor. It is not so much precisely what you do but why you have done it and what you have both given to it and gained from it.

Applicants could legitimately ask whether any factors, apart from the strength of the UCAS application form, enter into the selection for interview. It used to be customary at many medical schools (a tradition by no means confined to them) for the children of graduates of the school or of staff to be offered an interview, but that has now been abandoned out of conviction that the selection process must be and be seen to be open and, as far as can be, scrupulously fair.

Unsolicited letters of recommendation are a sensitive matter. Factual information additional to the UCAS confidential report is occasionally important and is welcome from any source. For example, one applicant had left another medical school in his first term against the advice of his dean to work to support his mother and younger brother. Three years later, when the family was on its feet and he wanted to reapply to medical school, he was under a cloud for having given up his place. The UCAS form did not tell the full story; and a note from the family doctor was most helpful in giving the full background to a courageous and self-sacrificing young man. Some other unsolicited letters add only the information that an applicant is either well connected or has good friends, and it is difficult to see why such applicants should be given an advantage over those whose friends do not feel it proper to canvass.

It is not only unsolicited testimonials that recommend in glowing terms. How could any dean resist the angel described thus by her headmaster:

> The charm of her personal character defies analysis. She is possessed by all the graces and her noble qualities impress everybody. She has proved the soul of courtesy and overlying all her virtues is sound common sense. She has always been mindful of her obligations and has fulfilled her responsibilities and duties as a prefect admirably well. Amiable and industrious, she appears to have a spirit incapable of boredom and her constructive loyalty to the school, along with her unfailing good nature, has won her the high esteem and admiration of staff and contemporaries alike. We recommend her warmly as a top drawer student.

A "top drawer" student indeed – and a top drawer headmaster.

When to apply

All UCAS forms for applicants to medicine must be received by 15th October at the latest, so get on with it as early as possible. Late applications are rarely even considered and almost never successful.

In principle a year's break between school and university is a good thing. The year is particularly valuable if used to experience the discipline and, often, the drudgery of earning a living from relatively unskilled work. It can provide insights for students (most of whom come from relatively well-off families) into the everyday life and thinking of the community which will provide most of their patients in due course and may be very different from their own background. There is no need for such work to be in the setting of health care; in fact much is to be said for escaping from the environment of doctors and hospitals.

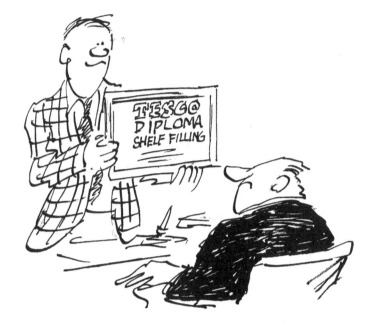

If the earnings of these months are then used to discover something of different cultures abroad that is a bonus. Alternatively, you may work abroad through Project Trust, Gap Projects, Operation Raleigh, or other similar organisations. But just being a year older, more experienced, and more mature is, in itself, helpful to the discipline and motivation of study and especially useful when you are faced with patients. In practice, short-term employment may, unfortunately, be difficult to find but there are few places where work of some description cannot be obtained if a student is prepared to do anything legal, however menial. Settling down to academic work again after a year off can be a problem, but it is not insuperable if the motivation and self-discipline are there. If commitment has evaporated after a year's break, better to have discovered early than late; better to drop out before starting rather than to waste a place that another could use and to waste your own time, which could better be channelled elsewhere.

A practical dilemma arises for those planning a year off over whether to apply for deferred entry before taking A levels or to apply with completed A levels early the year afterwards. Universities may be reluctant to commit themselves a year ahead to average applicants because the standard seems to be rising all the time. Outstanding applicants, however, should have no difficulty in arranging deferred entry before taking A levels, but it is worth checking the policy of schools in which you are interested before application. If you are not offered a deferred place apply early the next year and send a covering letter to the deans of your chosen medical schools asking for as early an interview as possible if you are planning to go abroad.

REMEMBER

- Each year about 17,000 home and EU students apply for 7500 places to read medicine in the UK.

- Over 700 places exist on shorter courses for graduates; mostly, but not entirely, science graduates.

- About 2300 overseas students apply for 550 places reserved for them at UK medical schools.

- Women comprise over half the applicants and entrants.

- Academic achievement is the strongest determinant in selection, but broader interests and achievements also count.

- It generally pays to apply as early as possible.

- Applications should be legible, honest, and, as far as possible, interesting.

- Use four choices for medicine; it is entirely reasonable to give a fifth and sixth to a non-medical option, but this is not compulsory.

- If you are planning a gap year, apply for a deferred entry rather than delay your application, and be prepared to discuss your plans for the year at interview.

6

Interviews

Academics and careers advisers debate the usefulness and fairness of an interview in the process for selecting future medical students and doctors. Those on the receiving end – the candidates – are unanimous in the belief that the interview is somewhere between daunting and dreadful. Some of the dread is fear of the unknown, as well as fear of being judged on what is little more than first impressions. Read on, and you may have some of those fears dispelled and be able to give yourself a better chance at creating a positive impression.

On a dull overcast day due for an imminent downpour, you step off the early morning train in your best new outfit, shoes polished, hair neatly brushed, clutching a copy of a newspaper in which you have just been reading an article about trendy new treatments for anxiety. As you approach the gates of the medical school and see the sign directing "Interview Candidates This Way" you wish you could remember any of the useful tips from that newspaper article; as it is you are so nervous you are no longer sure you can even remember your own name. It is not your first interview for a place at medical school, you had one last week. Although most of the details are lost in a haze of pounding heart-beats and sweaty palms, you are unable to rid yourself of the image of that professor's face when you dug yourself into a hole discussing the nutritional requirements of the Twa pygmies, a subject in which the sum of your knowledge was gleaned from the last 5 minutes of a late night documentary on BBC2. In what seemed like only half a minute, you are back at the railway station, on your way home, while the fearsome trio of interviewers dissect your inner being and decide your worth for that precious place at their medical school; your passport to their worthy profession. It feels like your life is in their hands.

SS

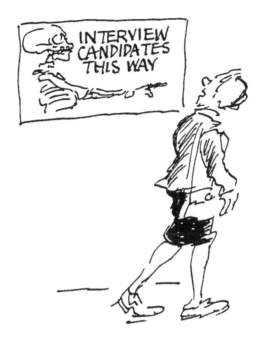

Most medical schools interview those students who seem the strongest on paper (through past achievements, predicted exam success, the confidential reference, and the student's own statements on the application form) and use the 15–20 minutes interview as a way of choosing between them. The remaining schools interview smaller numbers such as mature students, in an attempt to assess motivation and circumstances more fully.

The purpose

In general, the interview is an opportunity to test the students' awareness of what they are letting themselves in for, both at medical school and as a doctor. This can range from the impact of medicine on personal life to how medicine relates to the society it serves. It also allows the interviewers to explore whether applicants can communicate effectively, can think a problem through with logic and reason, and are speaking for themselves and not regurgitating well rehearsed answers which teachers and parents have thought up for them; it also reveals some of the qualities above and beyond academic ability which are desirable in a caring profession such as compassion and a sense of humour. Occasionally, a student who seems outstanding on paper can seem so lacking in motivation, insight, or humanity that he or she loses an offer which would otherwise have seemed a certainty. Likewise, the interview can allow students who seem equal on their Universities' and Colleges' Admissions Services (UCAS) forms to make their own case either through special circumstances or by a shining performance.

The panel

The interview panels differ in style and substance between schools but typically consist of three or four members of staff and often a student. The panel is a mixture of basic scientists, hospital consultants, and general practitioners, one of whom, often the senior admissions tutor, will take the chair. Members of panels attend in an individual capacity and not as representatives of particular specialties. They know that medicine offers a wide range of career opportunities, that most doctors will end up looking after patients but not all do, that more will work outside hospitals than in, and that both the training and the job itself are demanding physically and emotionally. They also know that whatever their final occupation doctors need to make decisions, deal with uncertainty, communicate effectively and compassionately with patients and colleagues alike as well as maintaining academic standards. The aim is not to pick men and women for specific tasks but to train wise, bright, humane, rounded individuals who will find their niche somewhere in medicine. The format may be formal, with the interview conducted in traditional fashion across a large table, or more informal, sitting in comfortable chairs around a coffee table by the fireside. The tenor of the interview, however, depends much more on the style of questioning; no matter how soft the armchairs they can still feel decidedly uncomfortable if you are made to feel like you are being grilled and about to be eaten for breakfast.

Dress and demeanour

Although the interview is a chance to be yourself and sell yourself, there are certain codes of conduct that even the most individual or eccentric candidate should be encouraged to heed. Rightly or wrongly first impressions count, and so what you wear matters. Dress smartly and comfortably and make an effort to look as presentable as you would expect from a mature professional. If your usual style of clothing is rather off beat, then perhaps for once it may be wise to let your tongue make any statements about your individuality rather than your all-in-one leather number and preference for multiple face piercing.

Nothing is more of a turn-off to interviewers than someone who is full of himself (or herself!) and seems to be finding it hard to accept that his offer is not a formality. On the other hand, an obviously talented and caring student whose modesty and nerves get the better of him and who fails to give the panel any reasons at all to give him an offer is almost as frustrating. The key is balance. When asked to blow your own trumpet, make it sound like a melodious fugue not a ship's fog horn. The best way to learn how to achieve this delicate balance is by practice. Many schools will be able to organise mock interviews, which can be useful, but often the more specific points relating to entering medical school can be best thought through by enlisting the help of your local family doctor or a family friend who is a doctor or by talking to anyone experienced in interviewing or being interviewed in any context or by asking the advice of people who have themselves recently been through it when you visit the medical schools on open days or tours.

The conversation

Almost anything can be asked. It would be advisable to have thought about such things as Why medicine? Why here? Why now? You should be able to show you have a realistic insight into the life of a doctor, and this is often best achieved by relating personal experience of spending some time with a doctor in hospital or general practice or, for example, by voluntary work in an old people's home or with children with special needs. Some panels put great store by your showing them how much you can achieve when you put your mind to it and will want to discuss your expedition to Nepal, your work on the school magazine, your musical or sporting successes. Remember to keep a copy of your UCAS form personal statement to read before you go into your interview. It is very often used as a source for questions and it can be embarrassing if you appear not to remember what you wrote. Even more importantly, do not invent interests or experience, as you may get caught out. One candidate at interview recently struggled through his interview after he was asked about the voluntary work at a local nursing home which he put on his form and replied: "I haven't actually got round to doing it yet, but I'd like to". He was not offered a place.

It is often sensible to have kept in touch with current affairs and developments in research. This is particularly relevant if the medical school has a strong interest in a research topic which has a high media profile. By reading a good quality daily newspaper you will greatly assist your ability to provide informed comment on issues of the moment. One candidate at interview cited the strong research background as a reason for applying to that school, and when asked to discuss which research at the school impressed him he replied: "Fleming's discovery of penicillin". He knew he had not done himself any favours when the dean replied: "Could you not perhaps think of anything a little more recent than 1928?"

With contentious issues such as ethics or politics, candidates will be neither criticised nor penalised for holding particular views but will be expected to be capable of explaining their case. Specific questions on subjects such as abortion, religion, or party politics are discouraged, but if they are likely to cause personal professional dilemmas it is reasonable and sensible to have thought about them and to be able to discuss how you would approach resolving such issues. Candidates with special circumstances, especially mature students, should be fully prepared for the interview panel to concentrate on particularly relevant factors such as whether they can afford to support themselves during the course, rigorous testing of their motivation, and questioning of the reasons behind their decision to enter the medical profession.

It is usual for the panel to offer an opportunity for the candidate to ask questions. A current student at the school sitting in on the interview can often be useful in answering the candidate's questions. Make sure if you do ask a question that you do not spoil an otherwise successful interview by asking a question which simply indicates that you have failed to read the prospectus thoroughly or which has no direct bearing on your entry to or time at medical school. It is perfectly acceptable, when asked if you have any questions, to say something along the lines: "No thank you, the student who showed me round answered all the questions I had".

Offers

An offer made to a candidate who has already achieved the minimum academic requirement is unconditional. All candidates who have already attained the minimum grades at first attempt cannot automatically receive a place because far more applicants will achieve this than the school can take. Offers are made on all round merit as can best be assessed on all the evidence.

If examinations have yet to be taken an offer is conditional on the candidate achieving the required grades at first attempt. Occasionally a student who seems in need of an incentive may be given a higher target but would normally be accepted with the minimum. Sometimes a lower than normal offer is made to reduce the pressure on a candidate working under exceptional circumstances. If exams are being retaken, most medical schools will expect higher than normal targets to be reached.

Finally, applicants must remember that achievement of minimum grades does no more than qualify them to enter the real competition. No level of exam success gives entitlement to a place without necessary consideration of the other factors important to being a doctor, an assessment of which is the whole basis for calling applicants to interview. Many more candidates can achieve the required grades than can possibly be taken under the fixed quota system which exists for the training of doctors. All medical schools try very hard to be fair but a number of able applicants will inevitably be disappointed.

REMEMBER

- Most medical schools interview all applicants to whom they make an offer.

- Usually a panel of three to five people – doctors, lecturers, and often a student observer – will be present.

- The interview will usually last 10–20 minutes, giving you time to settle into it – the interviewers know that you will be nervous, but try to relax and show yourself at your best.

- The major purpose of an interview is to test your awareness about the course and the career, and to discover whether you can think and reason for yourself.

- To prepare for the day read the prospectus thoroughly, read up on current relevant issues in the health section of a daily newspaper, arrange some practice interviews and be prepared to elaborate on what you wrote on your application form.

- On the day, dress smartly and comfortably, arrive in plenty of time, speak up clearly, and do not ask questions that have no direct bearing on entry to, or time at, medical school.

- Offers will be unconditional if the academic requirements have already been met, or for most applicants will be conditional on achieving target grades at the first attempt.

- All medical schools try hard to be fair but some able applicants will inevitably be disappointed.

7

Medical school: the early years

The first few weeks at medical school are bewildering. On top of all the upheaval of finding your feet in a new place, finding new friends, finding the supermarket, and finding that your bed does not miraculously make itself, you will find yourself at the beginning of a course that will mould the rest of your life. Ahead there are new subjects to study, a whole new language to learn, a new approach to seeing problems, new experiences and challenges, thrills and spills, ups and downs, laughter and tears. You are now at university, you are a medical student and you are on your way to being a doctor.

Until recently the undergraduate medical course had remained largely unaltered for decades, having slowly and steadily evolved over centuries of medical learning. All that has had to change in the past decade as the structure of the traditional course came face to face with the strains of modern medicine. The explosion of scientific knowledge, the unstoppable advances in technology, the ever-developing complexity of clinical practice, and changing health-care provision have all added to the tremendous demands on tomorrow's doctors.

At the same time there has been a reaction against the soaring dominance of modern science over old-fashioned art in medicine, technical capability over wise restraint, and process over humanity. A growing concern (not necessarily justified) that preoccupation with the diagnostic and therapeutic potential of molecular biology will obscure the patient as a whole person, a person who so often simply does not feel well for relatively trivial and unscientific reasons, and probably only needs to be listened to and encouraged to take responsibility for his or her own health. A fear that health-care teams under pressure from every direction may give the impression that they have forgotten how to care in the fullest sense – and, worse still, may indeed lose sight of the humanity of medicine.

The Prince of Wales put his finger on the issue in a "Personal View" in the *British Medical Journal*, writing "Many patients feel rushed and confused at seeing a different doctor each time … and many health-care professionals feel frustrated and dissatisfied at being unable to deliver the quality of care they would like in today's overstretched service".

There has also been a reaction against the traditionally closed mind of the medical profession towards complementary and alternative medicine, partly because of dissatisfaction with the fragmentation of conventional medicine and partly because of the effects of relentless pressure on doctors. As some patients derive benefit from unorthodox medicine (often when traditional medicine has failed) – however obscure the mechanism of the benefit may be – doctors need to be informed about such therapies and the evidence, such as it is, for their effectiveness. As the Prince of Wales observed in his "Personal View": "It would be a tragic loss if traditional human caring had to move to complementary medicine, leaving orthodox medicine with just

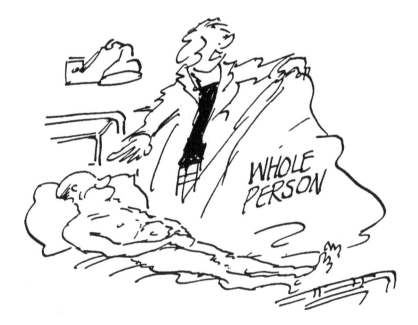

the technical management of disease". At the end of the day, it may well be that the greatest benefit of complementary therapies derives from the therapist being able to give more time to listening to the patient. Be that as it may, it is clearly in the patient's interest to "create a more inclusive system that incorporates the best and most effective of both complementary and orthodox medicine … choice where appropriate, and the best of both worlds whenever it is possible".

Recommendations published by the General Medical Council (GMC) in 2002 provided a new impetus to the introduction of a new medical curriculum. Less emphasis was put on absorbing facts like a sponge and more on thinking: on listening, analysing, questioning, problemsolving, explaining, and involving the patient in his or her own care; more emphasis on the patient as a whole in his or her human setting. The biological and behavioural basis of medicine in most medical schools now focuses on "need to know and understand". Oxford and Cambridge remain perfectly reasonable exceptions, having retained a strongly and intrinsically medical science centred curriculum in the first 3 years. The GMC encourages diversity within the curriculum and students should carefully consider which sort of curriculum would best inspire their mind, heart, and enthusiasm.

You can usually get a flavour of how the course is delivered at each school by reading the curriculum and students' views section on the medical schools' web sites (see Appendix 5) or in their prospectuses.

Nevertheless, at most universities the traditionally separate scientific and clinical aspects of the course have become very substantially integrated to prevent excited and enthusiastic students becoming disillusioned in the first 2 years with what understandably seemed to be divorced from real patients and real lives, from clinical relevance and clinical understanding.

The most recent development in undergraduate medical education has been that of the Medical School Charter from the Council of Heads of Medical Schools and BMA medical students (see Appendix 1). Launched in 2006 this document enlists the rights and responsibilities of medical students in part one and medical schools in part two and represents a 'contract' that students sign on enrolling at medical school. To date, it has been adopted by University of East Anglia, Leicester, Southampton, Aberdeen and Cardiff, with more medical schools expected to join in the future. The charter will be reviewed every 2 years.

The subjects, systems and topics

Most first-year students begin with a foundation course covering the fundamental principles of the basic medical sciences. These include anatomy – the structure of the human body, including cell and tissue biology and embryology, the process of development; physiology – the normal functions of the body; biochemistry – the chemistry of body processes, with increasing amounts of molecular biology and genetics; pharmacology – the properties and metabolism of drugs within the body; psychology and sociology – the basis of human behaviour and the placing of health and illness in a wider context; and basic pathology – the general principles underlying the process of disease.

As the general understanding of the basics increases, the focus of the teaching often then moves from parallel courses in each individual subject to integrated interdepartmental teaching based on body systems – such as the respiratory system, the cardiovascular system, or the locomotor system – and into topics such as development and aging, infection and immunity, and public health and epidemiology.

In the systems approach the anatomy, physiology, and biochemistry of a system can be looked at simultaneously, building up knowledge of the body in a steady logical way. As time and knowledge progress the pathology and pharmacology of the system can be studied, and the psychological and sociological aspects of related illnesses are considered.

Often the normal structure and function can best be understood by illustrating how it can go wrong in disease, and so clinicians are increasingly involved at an early stage; this has an added advantage of placing the science into a patient-focused context, making the subject more relevant and stimulating for would-be doctors. It also allows for early contact with patients to take place in the form of clinical demonstrations or, for example, in a project looking at chronic disease in a general practice population or on a hospital ward.

In some medical schools, such as Manchester and Liverpool, practically all the learning in the early years is built around clinical problems that focus all the different dimensions of knowledge needed to understand the illness, the patient, and the management.

The teaching and the teachers

The teaching of these subjects usually takes the form of lectures, laboratory practicals, demonstrations, films, tutorials and projects, and, increasingly, computer-assisted interactive learning programmes; even virtual reality is beginning to find its uses in teaching medical students.

The teaching of anatomy in particular has undergone great change. Dissection of dead bodies (cadavers) has been replaced in most schools by increased use of closed circuit television and demonstrations of prosected specimens and an ever-improving range of synthetic models. Preserved cadavers make for difficult dissection, especially in inexperienced if enthusiastic hands, and, although many regarded the dissecting room as an important initiation for the young medical student, fortunately much of the detail needed for surgical practice is revised and extended later by observing and assisting at operations and during postgraduate training. Much more useful to general clinical practice is the increased teaching of living and radiological anatomy. In living anatomy, which is vital before trying to learn how to

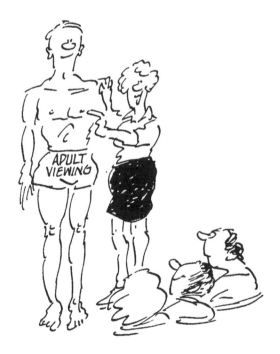

examine a patient, the surface markings of internal structures are learnt by using each other as models. This makes for a fun change from a stuffy lecture theatre as willing volunteers (and there are always one or two in every year) strip off to their smalls while some blushing colleague draws out the position of their liver and spleen with a felt tip marker pen.

Similarly, with the technological advances in imaging parts of the body with X-rays, ultrasound, computed tomography, magnetic resonance imaging, radionucleotide scans, and the like, and their subsequent use in both diagnosis and treatment, the need to have a basic understanding of anatomy through radiology has never been greater.

Practical sessions in other subjects, especially physiology and pharmacology, often involve students performing simple tests on each other under supervision. Memorable afternoons are recalled in the lab being tipped upside down on a special revolving table while someone checked my blood pressure or peddling on an exercise bike at 20 kilometre per hour for half an hour with a long air pipe in my mouth and a clip on my nose while my vital signs were recorded by highly entertained friends or recording the effect on the colour of my urine of eating three whole beetroots, feeling relieved not to be the one who had to test the effects of 20 fish oil capsules. As well as the performing of the experiments, the collation and analysis of the data and the researching and writing up of conclusions is seen as central to the exercise, and so students may find themselves being introduced to teaching in information technology, effective use of a library, statistics, critical reading of academic papers, and data handling and presentation skills.

The teaching of much of the early parts of the course is carried out by basic medical scientists, most of whom are not medically qualified but who are specialist researchers in their subject. Few have formal training in teaching but despite this the quality of the teaching is generally good and the widespread introduction of student evaluation of their teachers is pushing up standards even further. Small group tutorials play an important part in supplementing the more formal lectures, particularly when learning is centred around a problemsolving approach, with students working through clinical-based problems to aid the understanding of the system or topic being studied at that time. The tutorial system is also an important anchor point for students who find the self-discipline of much of the learning harder than the spoon-feeding they may have become used to at school.

Students may also have an academic tutor or director of studies or a personal tutor, or both, a member of staff who can act as a friend and adviser. The success or failure of such a system depends on the individuals concerned, and many students prefer to obtain personal advice from sympathetic staff members they encounter in their day-to-day course rather than seeking out a contrived adviser with whom they have little or no natural contact. In some schools, most notably in Oxbridge, the college-based tutor system is much more established and generally plays a more important personal and academic part.

Links are sometimes also set up between new students and those in older years; these "link friends", "mentors", or "parents" can often be extremely useful sources of information on a whole range of issues from which textbooks to buy to which local general practitioner to register with and useful tips on how to study for examinations, and of course numerous suggestions on how to spend what little spare time you can scrape together.

In every school there will be a senior member of staff, a sub-dean or director of medical education, who oversees the whole academic programme and can follow the progress of individuals and offer a guiding hand where needed.

As students progress other topics are added into the course. Most schools provide first-aid training for their students, and a choice of special study modules (SSMs) are offered each year to encourage students to spend some time studying in breadth or depth an area which interests them and in which they can develop more knowledge and understanding. Early patient contact is encouraged; sometimes through schemes which link a junior student with a ward where small group teaching takes place or through projects or simply by gaining experience of the work of other staff, such as nurses, health visitors, physiotherapists, and occupational therapists; or time can be spent just talking to patients and relatives. Some schools begin a module in the first year which introduces aspects of clinical training, ideally in the setting of general practice, with the same doctor every week or two for 1 or 2 years. The supervised learning includes skills such as history taking and clinical examination or the interpretation of results of clinical investigations.

In the early part of some courses students may be introduced to a local family with whom they will remain in contact for the duration of their time as a student. Such attachment schemes, which are often organised by general practice departments, are designed to give students a realistic experience of the effects on people of events such as childbirth, bereavement, financial hardship, or ill health from a perspective which few would otherwise encounter.

It is difficult to get the true feel of being in the early years of medical training from the rather dry description of the course, so let two students at that stage themselves describe a typical week in their lives on different preclinical medicine courses.

A week on a problem-based learning course – Manchester

Thursday

Yes, Thursday is the start of the week as far as we're concerned in Manchester. At least that's when we start each new case.

The idea behind problem-based learning (PBL) is that we use real clinical problems (or cases) as the main stimulus for our learning. Each week we have a new case to study; understanding the background to the problem itself and exploring aspects related to it. Nobody tells us what we "need" to know, we must decide for ourselves which information is important to learn and understand. At first, like everybody, I found it difficult to adjust to this new way of learning – I was used to the spoon-fed process at school which helped me pass my A levels. I found it quite daunting and challenging to make up my own learning objectives and search out the information for myself. Once I got used to it, however, it became a really enjoyable way to study medicine. I found myself actually wanting to spend time in the library or in hospital to find the answers to my questions. I quickly found out that there is no need to rote learn all the muscle attachments of the bones in the hand or every single anatomical feature of the femur. I learnt to discriminate between useless information and useful information – for example, how antidepressants work or the functions of the stomach.

In the past, medics on traditional courses spent their first 2 years trying to cram textbooks of information into their heads and usually hating every minute of it, desperately waiting for the clinical years. If you ask them how much information they retained after their preclinical exams were over they'll find it difficult to admit that they forgot nearly everything straightaway! By using the PBL method to learn medicine the information we learn now is more likely to be retained in the future, long after our exams when we're doctors on the wards. I discovered that it's a very satisfying way to learn medicine as I am constantly solving cases and applying my knowledge to real-life situations. My motivation to learn is increased and because I actually want and like to learn I find it easier to understand and remember what I read about. It's one thing being able to learn facts and principles, it's quite another to apply them in real life. PBL helps us to learn the skills necessary to do this – skills that we must learn to be good doctors.

In Manchester, the first 2 years are divided into four semesters. Each semester has a title – for example, Nutrition and Metabolism, Cardiorespiratory Fitness. This semester I am studying "Abilities and Disabilities", and it involves learning mainly about the brain, nervous system, muscles, and bones.

At 10 a.m. I have a theatre event. This usually means going into the lecture theatre (hence the name!) to listen to a lecture, but sometimes we'll watch a video or take part in a clinical demonstration. The lectures are usually interactive too, and we're encouraged to ask questions or participate in discussion. The theatre event this morning introduced us to aspects of that week's case by giving us an overview of how the eye works. The patient in the case this week is followed from childhood (when she has a squint) through to old age (when her eyesight deteriorates, partly due to disease).

Afterwards I decided to go to the library for a couple of hours to read up before my first discussion group. Each week we study the case with our tutor group (consisting of about 12–15 students).We have 3 1-hour meetings in the week to work through the case. This week, Mary is assigned the role of chairperson and Mike is scribe. The chairperson tries to keep the discussion on track (and keep us under control!) whereas the scribe has the job of writing the important points down during the session and typing them up. We rotate the two jobs each week so everyone has a chance. Each group has two tutors who are always present but usually do not take part in the discussion unless we ask them a specific question. One tutor is a basic medical scientist and the other is a clinician. The tutors are there to facilitate our discussion and will interrupt us only if we go off on a tangent. The clinician is also there as our main link to hospital and will invite us in to have small group teaching on the wards or will make it possible for us to come in pairs to shadow other doctors on shifts. In my first year I chose to spend a Saturday night in accident and emergency. Unfortunately (or fortunately!), it was not the *Casualty/ER* scenario I expected, and two drunks and a regular were the only ones to come in during the entire 12-hour shift.

We usually read through the case in the first session, defining things we don't understand, using clues in the case to decide what we need to learn about, and dividing up the tasks between us. We form learning objectives based on the case itself, which means that we cover anatomy, physiology, biochemistry, pharmacology, psychology, etc., altogether instead of each subject being learned separately. I've found that this method of learning medicine, the "systems-based" method, gives me a more complete picture and I'm able to connect up the anatomy, physiology, etc., of an organ better and remember how they are related to each other. It also means that we understand disease processes more thoroughly and that we're encouraged to look at the patient as a whole person within society not just as an illness.

Friday

I didn't have to be in for dissection until 11 a.m. We have 2 hours of dissection every week when we get hands-on experience of the body and primarily discuss anatomy with a tutor in our tutor groups. Today we dissected the eye and the orbit of the brain of our cadaver. The first time I saw the cadaver was a moment I'll remember forever, and I think dissection is one of the most interesting times of the week, the only thing I don't like is the smell! We also use this time to do living anatomy and look at X-ray pictures and body scans.

Just had time to grab a sandwich from the coffee bar before the theatre event at 1 p.m. This time it was a demonstration and video about how the eye detects colour, especially in the dark. It was really good fun, and we experimented with optical illusions. Finished again at 3 p.m. and went to the library for an hour to learn more about colour vision but found it difficult to focus on the textbook at first since my eyes were still suffering from the optical illusions.

Weekend

I spent most of the weekend in the library, working on the case. Except for Saturday morning when I played in a mixed hockey match against Edinburgh medics. Medicine takes up a large part of my life but I always manage to find time to do other things.

Monday

Early start for computers at 9 a.m. We have 2 hours of computing class every week. We also learn about statistics during that time and how to carry out statistical procedures using the computer. I didn't do statistics at school but it's not a disadvantage since we are taken through things step by step. It's the same with computing so that even if you've never even switched one on before, it soon becomes possible to produce spreadsheets and data analyses.

At 11 a.m. I have histology class. We also have 2 hours of histology a week. We work through the lesson in pairs with the help of tutors. Depending on the case, I sometimes find myself spending longer in the lab to make sure I've seen everything that I'm supposed to see down the microscope. Although it can be fascinating this is not my favourite medical pastime.

That was it for the day and I was able to take my time over lunch. In the afternoon Lucy and I headed across to the Manchester Royal Infirmary. We eventually found the ophthalmology department and introduced ourselves to the nurses and met the consultant as arranged. We were able to see five patients during the 3 hours we were there, and it really opened my eyes to the treatments possible.

Tuesday

From 9 to 11 a.m. we had lab work. This is the time when we learn how to carry out certain examinations or procedures, everything from blood pressure measurement to drug dilutions. This week we learnt how to examine the eye with an ophthalmoscope and carry out an eye test like you have done at the opticians. It was more complicated than it seemed, and it took me and my partner Toby the entire 2 hours to get through everything.

At noon we had our second discussion group. Lucy and I gave an account about what we'd seen on the ward, and Farid gave a presentation on how laser treatments work to improve eyesight. We discussed the case but realised there were still some aspects to it we didn't understand. Some people were assigned specific things to find out for tomorrow's session. We also agreed to go out for a group meal tomorrow night! We do this about twice each semester so we have some time to socialise together as a group.

At 3 p.m. we had another theatre event, this one was about eye surgery and the techniques they use – it was quite gruesome. At the end of the lecture we had a feedback session. Each semester we're asked to give our opinions on how the course is going and any improvements that we think should be made. We fill in lots of questionnaires about everything, from the books we use in the library to what we think of our tutors. The staff are really good and although PBL is now well established in its third year, they are still willing to make changes and genuinely listen to our problems. Students are actively involved in all faculty committees too. We finished at 4 p.m. but I went to the computer lab to use one of the computerassisted learning (CAL) programmes. I like using them because they're more interactive than textbooks; they usually have quizzes so I can test myself at the end.

Wednesday

At 10 a.m. we had our final discussion session about the case. It was quite a good session since we managed to tie up nearly all our loose ends and still had time to talk about the social issues that the case raised. Our clinical tutor gave us a clinical perspective on the case and told us a few of his experiences too.

The good thing about working in groups is that it helps us to develop our communication skills. We are always having to explain our theories and listen to each other, which means we get very good at talking about medicine. It is good preparation for us as future doctors as we'll have to do this constantly with patients. I've become very good at working in a team too – an invaluable skill to have as a doctor.

That evening we had a group night out and went for a curry. One of the best things about PBL is that you really get to know the people in your group very well because you work together as a team. You go through a lot together, and the groups are small enough to allow you to work closely with everyone during the semester.

I really enjoy studying medicine PBL style. It teaches you important and essential skills for being a doctor as well as being brilliant fun.

C-MB

A week on a problem-based learning course – Bart's and the London

Here at Bart's and the London (BL) our first 2 years are split using a systems-based approach. There are six modules set in this way throughout the year, cardiorespiratory, metabolism, brain and behaviour, human development, human sciences and public health, and locomotor. These are also interspersed with two selected study modules in the year, where we have a number of choices for what we want to study over a 2-week period.

Our course is grounded in problem-based learning (PBL) within a "learning landscape" that involves anatomy specimens, imaging of the particular area we are working on at the time, computer-based learning sessions, and practical and clinical skills sessions where we learn to examine each body system. There is also allocated "self-directed learning" (SDL) time in order to go away and read around the subjects which have arisen within PBL.

Every 2 weeks we have "medicine in society" or MedSoc, where in the first year we are based at a GP surgery and in the second year in the community or a hospital setting. This gives us the opportunity to meet, and talk with patients, and practice skills which we have learnt in other sessions, whilst discussing problems with our allocated doctors and other MedSoc tutors.

Right now I'm in my second year. The current topic is Human Sciences and Public Health and, though it's not my favourite module in the world, it's an important aspect of medicine. It covers research and clinical trials, along with statistics and how to interpret them. We also cover ethics and law within medicine, bringing up important issues which we will, no doubt, encounter throughout our careers. We study public health and sociology – the motivation of patients and how to make treatments more effective for them and their lives. This week we have several PBL sessions: one on sudden infant death syndrome (SIDS) and its contributing factors/causes; another on a diabetic patient and the way in which cultural issues, lifestyle factors, and health beliefs play a part in his disease; another on old age, illness and society, and an epidemiology review; and a final one on a man who suffered a heart attack, considering the link between a stressful job, a smoking habit, and disease. We also have lectures on support networks, stress, personality and illness and gender differences in health. On top of all this its RAG week! RAG stands for raising and giving for charity, and here at Bart's and the London it is a very big week in the calendar. Since I'm on the committee it is also a very tiring one, involving early starts, keeping up with work, and late nights. However, it is one of the most rewarding weeks here too, as we are the top collectors out of all the London medical schools. Tonight for example is the RAG Dental Beer Race. I am really looking forward to it and am hoping that I won't get too many odd looks painted orange and dressed as an oompa-lumpa!

Since it is RAG week and there is so much to be done, the older years help out the first and second years with their PBLs so that it doesn't all get too much. There is a lot of integration between the years in terms of social and other extracurricular activities and we get to know everyone, not just those in our own year – it also means we get a lot of advice and help if we need it. It is a brilliant support network.

I love studying medicine, and the people who are part of that. It might be one heck of a challenge sometimes, but there are always moments which make you realise why you do it and make you see the bigger picture – and besides, where's the reward without a challenge?!

SV

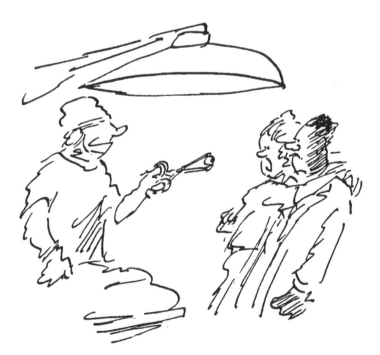

Communication skills

The teaching of communication skills to medical students has improved greatly across the board in recent years, largely in response to public demand. Patients want to know more about their condition and to have more involvement in the decisions, for instance about treatment options, which affect their lives. The skills needed to communicate well with patients are often not fully appreciated, and many, including well-established doctors think it is something you either have or do not have.

While it is true that some doctors do have a natural flair for the right bedside manner and know instinctively when to hold a hand or when a moment of quiet reflection is appropriate, many of the skills can in fact be learnt quite easily. Such skills are not just about explaining procedures and breaking bad news but also about how and when to keep quiet and listen, to ask the right questions in the right way, drawing out the patient's story, which allows you to make an accurate diagnosis and formulate a suitable management plan, as well as earning trust and showing empathy. Much of this teaching is done in small groups and uses actors' role playing patients with fellow students watching on television monitors. This type of training is also a compulsory part of postgraduate training in general practice, so the practice early on is time doubly well spent. Let a former student describe her experiences of communication skills training.

Communication skills

You will be spending the rest of your prospective career talking to patients so it's nice to be able to do it well – indeed it's one of the major ways in which your medical skills are judged. To this end, the communication skills teaching is designed to give you a few pointers as to how to handle various patient scenarios so that you and the patient go away happy (and less liable to sue!).

There is a small group of students, a doctor, psychologist, and a TV/video at each session. You are in the room next door with an actor and a video camera to keep you company. Before it starts, all you can think of are your friends watching you on TV next door in this totally artificial situation and how stupid it all seems! But then the actor arrives playing your patient and you're away. They might be trying to tell you about their piles or of "trouble down below, Doctor". They may be a shy, retiring nun or the Marquis de Sade, anything is fair game. There are various scenarios and patients that the actors can play, and they are invariably superb. You forget it's all a sham and that your friends are next door watching you on TV.

A particular favourite that you are asked to do is explain to a patient (actor) a special test he or she needs to have done and what it will be like for him or her. The old chestnut is endoscopy. This usually leads to some wonderful descriptions of TV cameras being forced down the unfortunate patient's throat which, judging by their aghast expressions, seems to conjure up images of the cameraman, floor manager, and producer going down to have a look, too! The most difficult to explain are tests involving the injection of a harmless radioactive isotope. On at least one occasion the patient left the room convinced his hair would fall out and his skin peel and blister in a most Chernobyl-esque manner!

After the consultation you go back next door and receive comments from those watching. Emphasis is put on your good points as well as your goofs, so it boosts your confidence (that's half the trick in good communication) for dealing with real patients, as well as raising your awareness of the possible pitfalls. Invaluable skills are learnt, which past students, now doctors, say they are still using on the wards now.

LJ

Intercalated honours degrees

An increasing number of students are choosing to spend an extra year studying for an honours degree during the medical course. This is usually a Bachelor of Science (BSc) or Bachelor of Medical Science (BMedSci) and can usually be taken from the end of the second year to the beginning of the final year, depending on the design of the course and the exact nature of the subject being studied. These degrees can either have a more basic science emphasis – for example, extending study from a SSM in neurosciences or neonatal physiology – or if it is taken later in the course some schools offer clinical science-related degrees. This extra year of study is often the only opportunity an undergraduate has to experience front-line scientific research; besides the subject knowledge gained, it is a unique chance to develop skills in research and laboratory techniques, and writing scientific papers. Occasionally there are opportunities for a much broader range of study encompassing humanities such as history of medicine or modern languages. There are numerous grants and scholarships available from schools and research funds to assist with the expense of this additional year to cover living expenses if not tuition fees. Despite the extra expense the number of students seeing the advantages of making the sacrifices needed to take up this valuable opportunity is continuing to grow.

There are several notable exceptions to the general design of the intercalated degrees being outlined here. At St Andrew's University the student takes a 3-year (or 4 if an honours degree) preclinical course leading to a BSc in Medical Sciences and then usually transfers to clinical studies at Manchester University. At both Imperial College and the Royal Free and University College London School of Medicine a 6-year course includes a modular BSc (Hons) as well as the MBBS. At Nottingham University, all students on the 5-year course are awarded a BMedSci if they successfully complete the first 3 years, which includes research-based project work.

The other main exceptions are the courses at Oxford and Cambridge, whose first 3 years lead to a Bachelor of Arts degree, in Medical Sciences at Cambridge and Physiological Sciences at Oxford.

Occasionally a student who has a particular research interest continues the BSc break in their medical course to complete a further 3 years of advanced research leading to the award of Doctor of Philosophy (PhD). Some medical schools such as Cambridge and University College, London, offer selected students a combined MB/PhD which is shorter than taking the two degrees separately.

Assessment

The variety and complexity of the courses offered by different medical schools are reflected in the numerous types of assessment used to check the progress of each student's learning. Attendance is not usually checked, but a student who is thought to be missing large amounts of the course should expect to be questioned by tutors and the senior tutor to discover whether there are any major problems with which the school may be able to help. Like most university courses the obligation to attend is the responsibility of the student, and it is salutary to note that poor course attendance, for whatever reason, corresponds highly with failing the early phases of the course.

Most schools use a mixture of continuous assessment of course work and major examinations at the end of terms or years, though the balance varies greatly. There are pros and cons of both systems, with students at schools where examinations play a larger part wishing that more credit were given to good work throughout the year rather than everything resting on their performance on one particular day. Students who undergo more continuous assessment, however, complain about the stresses and strains of frequent tests and projects, so it seems to be a case of "swings and roundabouts".

Around 5% of students fail to complete the course, most of these leaving at the end of the first year. This is most commonly due to a waning of motivation, the realisation of a wrong career choice, or, unfortunately, because of misjudgements of the amount of work necessary and a failure to organise their time effectively or because of the diversions of personal entanglements. A few fail their second or third year assessments, but students surviving this far have generally worked out what is required of them to qualify.

There is often a chance to resit examinations or resubmit unsatisfactory course work, but this is not to be recommended as it leads to extra work often at times when friends are away on vacations, sunning themselves on faraway beaches or earning much needed cash in holiday jobs. In exceptional circumstances, such as illness or bereavement, students may be allowed to resit a whole year, but this often has financial implications which may preclude some people. In any event, students who are experiencing difficulties are encouraged to discuss the problems with their tutor or another member of staff sooner rather than later.

Working hard, playing hard

On my first day at medical school the then president of the Royal College of Radiologists, Dr Oscar Craig, told the assembled mass of eager freshers, "this is the greatest day of your life". He continued, "Does it take great brains to become a doctor? I hate to disappoint you, but I don't think it does, you know. Does it take hard work and determination? … Like nothing else!"

Students who have gained a place at medical school have not only proved themselves bright enough to cope with the academic rigours of the course but have also usually shown exceptional interest or achievement in some other area or activity, often an activity requiring teamwork. It is usual then for medical schools to be hives of activity on the social scene, where clubs and societies abound providing sports fixtures, training sessions, plays and concerts, balls and discos, talks on this and that, and trips to here and there, all of which can lead to a wonderfully full life.

While the object of going to medical school is ultimately to train as a doctor, most students take full advantage of the chance to pursue their hobbies or try new ones, meet new friends, do new things, and generally do all the "growing up and finding yourself" things that students are supposed to do. The secret in all this is the fine balancing act between work and play. Each year a few potentially good doctors forget the real reason for their being at medical school, fail their examinations, and have to leave their friends and all that social life behind, not to mention having to find a new career. It is an unpleasant feeling seeing a good friend and colleague being asked to leave, so a great effort is made to encourage students to find the right balance so that medical schools train doctors who are both skilled at their job and also interesting and talented in other things; something they will cherish in later life.

REMEMBER

- Being a medical student, like any university student, is a complete change from being at school – you will have endless opportunities available to you but you will need to realise them for yourself.

- There is generally much less "spoon-feeding" and more self-directed learning, requiring self-motivation, determination and discipline, which some students find difficult at first.

- All medical courses now provide early clinical insights and problem-solving in addition to teaching the scientific and ethical basis of medicine.

- Courses range from the recognisably traditional at Oxford, Cambridge, and St Andrew's to substantially more integrated, problem-based approaches such as at Liverpool and Manchester.

- Several universities have introduced shorter (four year) courses for graduate students.

- A few universities award a science degree as an integral part of the medical course; most universities award a BSc or BMedSci degree for an optional, additional (intercalated) year.

- Assessment in the early years is by a variable mixture of continuous assessments and end of year examinations.

- Achieving the right balance between work and play can be a challenge for some new medical students, but most succeed.

- About 5% of students overall fail to complete the course, most in the first 2 years and they normally find fulfilling careers outside medicine.

8

Medical school: the later years

As the medical student progresses through into their third year and beyond, increasing amounts of time are spent in the various clinical teaching settings and less in the classroom. The white coat is donned, and the shiny new stethoscope is placed ostentatiously in the pocket, usually alongside numerous pocket-sized textbooks, pens, notepads, and sweet wrappers. Most students by now have some experience of listening and talking to patients and of the hospital wards. The sight of the ill patient in a bed does not come as the awful surprise it did to generations of medical students who spent their first 2 years cocooned in the medical school.

The style of teaching changes emphasis, becoming more of an apprentice-ship but retaining the academic backup of lectures, seminars, and particularly tutorials. More of the course is taught by clinical staff: consultants, general practitioners (GP), and junior doctors, often in small groups at the bedside, on dedicated teaching rounds or in tutorials, in the operating theatre, in the outpatient clinic, or general practice surgery. Teaching also takes place at clinical meetings or grand rounds and the firm's regular radiology meeting (when the week's X-ray pictures and scans are reviewed and discussed with a radiologist) and histopathology meeting (when the results of tissue biopsies and postmortem examinations are discussed). Some students find the change in the style of teaching frustrating as much time seems to be wasted hanging around waiting for teaching that never seems to happen. The registrar or consultant who is due to be teaching is often delayed in theatre with a difficult case or still has a queue of patients waiting in the outpatient clinic. Many of these doctors are fitting in their teaching commitments around an already punishing clinical workload, and so often a combination of better organisation by the schools and some initiative in self-directed learning from the students is all that is needed to extract the value from such a valuable educational source.

It may well be that with so much to learn, insufficient attention is given to the formation of attitudes. It is said that medical students have more appropriate attitudes to both patients and to others with whom they share care when they enter medical school than when they qualify as doctors. There may be more than a grain of truth in this. In the Bristol report, Professor Sir Ian Kennedy expressed the view that "the education and training of all health care professionals should be imbued with the idea of partnership … (with) … the patient … whereby the patient and the professional meet as equals". As far as mutual respect in teamwork is concerned, opportunities for learning together (multidisciplinary learning), both in the undergraduate and postgraduate years, are not fully exploited.

Much can be learned from reasonable complaints. A patient who had complained about the attitude of his surgeon was interviewed by another surgeon as part of a formal investigation into the complaint. The patient was pleased to find that the investigating surgeon was a complete contrast – "conversational, sympathetic, and informative; wide ranging and encouraged

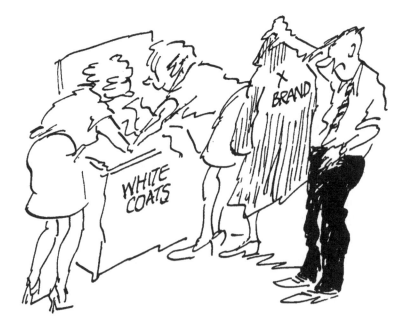

questions (with) a very human approach which inspired trust". As the complainant explained, the matter need never have reached the stage of formal complaint: all he had been seeking was "a small acceptance (from the first surgeon) that some of the procedures are inadequate and will be revised". Arrogance is something that students need to lose early in their training, if they have the misfortune to be afflicted by it; patients can do without it.

First patients

Stepping tentatively on to the ward for the first time, resplendent in my new white coat, I felt that the long awaited moment had arrived. "Clerking" involves taking a history from and examining the patient. We had been told that this process, which has been handed down from doctor to medical student for countless generations, enables the doctor to make 95% of the diagnosis (75% from the history and a further 20% from the examination – the last 5% comes from further investigations). This is why clerking has and will continue to be such a powerful tool in the hands of the clinician, though not necessarily in the hands of a junior clinical student.

On the first day of the junior course we learn how to take a thorough history. This involves an overall framework of "presenting complaint", "history of presenting complaint", "past medical history", "family history", "drug history", "social history", and "any other information". With practice it becomes possible to tailor the history taking to the individual.

Next comes the examination, something which opens up a veritable minefield for the inexperienced. When you perform a general examination every body system has to be inspected, palpated (lightly and deeply), percussed (examined by tapping with the fingers and listening to the pitch of the sound produced), and auscultated (listened to with a stethoscope). This is the theory but inevitably, either through incompetence or sheer bad luck, it is almost impossible to perform a perfect examination on every patient: some of the pulses are not felt or the enlarged liver does not seem that enlarged; whatever the sign of disease that causes such frustration by escaping the student, you can guarantee that the senior house officer will come along and find it within seconds!

The introduction to basic surgical techniques was one of the better activities organised for us during the junior clinical course. Armed with scalpels, sutures, forceps, and pigs' trotters the surgeons demonstrated the basic principles of stitching wounds and then let us loose on our own practice limbs. This was an excellent afternoon for the students, not least because it gave us the opportunity to do something incredibly practical that most of us had never done before. Having mastered (?) the mattress stitch, we moved on to the more cosmetically friendly subcuticular stitch, and I am sure we greatly impressed our surgical superiors with our manual dexterity!

The afternoon concluded with teaching us how to draw up and mix drugs with a syringe and how to inject them subcutaneously and intramuscularly (the intramuscular route was cleverly improvised with an orange).

My first firm was a series of firsts. First clerking of a patient – nerve racking as the whole scenario is new. I felt ill equipped and slightly obtrusive as I clumsily searched, questioned, and of course palpated and percussed my patient. The sense of relief as I parted the curtains and left the cubicle, history complete, was overwhelming.

First ward round – how I regretted not learning my anatomy better as in the words of our senior registrar I displayed "chasms of ignorance", only managing to redeem myself by the narrowest of margins.

First surgical operation – it was a real privilege to clerk a patient, then later watch and even assist in the operation and later still revisit the patient on the ward. Theatre also provided a superb way to learn by watching but also by the excellent active teaching of the surgeons.

First freedom – for the first time since entering medical school I was expected to decide for myself where to go to, what to learn, what to read, and to think more laterally and broadly than ever before.

First encounter with real patients with lives we are able to be part of for some small time – call us naive and overenthusiastic and we would agree. We are sure that some of the novelty will wear off after nights on take and unpleasant patients. Call us idealistic and we would agree and pray that it may be a comment levelled at us not just now as we experience our "firsts" but on until we experience our very "lasts". When idealism dies it is not replaced by realism but by cynicism and long may we be idealistic realists.

AH, SC

Meanwhile, at another medical school, another student was seeing a similar experience through somewhat different eyes.

First clinical "firm"

The first day as a clinical student is a little like the first time you have sex. There is a lot of anxiety and excitement for what often ends up as a disappointing and humiliating experience. At last an escape from lecture halls and seminar rooms; an end to being force fed mind numbing facts such as the course of the left recurrent laryngeal nerve or the intricacies of gluconeogenesis. I had a crisp white coat and smart matching shirt and tie. The finishing touch being a stethoscope slung casually around my neck. I had arrived, I looked fantastic, and I was IT.

I was attached to a firm run by a consultant whose fearsome reputation was unrivalled in the region. She had a moustache that Stalin would have been proud of and a personality to match. My fellow students were a real mixed bag; two rugby lads, two sloanes, a girly swot, a computer geek, and a goth! Most medical students wear a common uniform; boys in light blue shirts, stripy ties (preferably rugby ties), chinos (regulation length one inch too short), and either shiny, pointy shoes or those brown deck shoe things. Girls tend to opt for simple blouses with pretty necklines and floaty, flowery, shapeless skirts … invariably sensible and never fashionable.

Every aspect of being a clinical student combines in an attempt both to educate you and to expose you to the realities of being a junior doctor. The time is split between seeing patients on the wards, teaching sessions, sitting in clinics, and assisting in operating theatres. The day usually begins with a ward round. Medicine is like a huge machine; everyone has an allocated role; everyone is an essential moving part. The system works well if we all know our place and act according to our roles. The ward round reflects this system and demonstrates the hierarchy and tradition that exists in medicine. The consultant is the boss. His (or less commonly her) role is twofold. Firstly, to impart knowledge to the more junior members of the team (that is, everyone) in the form of witty and wise anecdotes and, secondly, to use derision, disapproval or old-fashioned humiliation on his or her juniors lest they forget their places.

Next in line are the registrars who are occasionally allowed to adopt the role of the consultant if he or she is otherwise engaged at the golf course/race course/Harley Street. Very rarely registrars are allowed to know something the consultant doesn't. There are strict limitations on what this information can be, but it generally involves very obscure areas of research that will never make it into the textbooks anyway! The senior house officers and house officers ensure the smooth running of the firm; taking notes, making lists, organising tests, and collecting results. They are also objects for ritual humiliation (that is, teaching) when the students are not around. Your role as a student is not difficult; laugh at the consultant's jokes, help out when needed, learn lots, and make great tea.

I was strangely reassured to find that ward rounds conformed to my preconceived idea of an all powerful consultant sweeping down the ward with an entourage of doctors and students following in order of decreasing seniority. Each student is allocated their own patients. On this particular day, my luck is in; the procession stops at the bedside of a young asthmatic man with a chest infection. He is not my patient. The student concerned steps forward, a little flushed and sweaty, but none-the-less does a good job of presenting her case and answers well under interrogation from the consultant. Her triumph, however, is short lived. It is revealed that she has not looked in the patient's sputum pot for 3 days. This is just short of a hanging offence on a respiratory firm!

There are a number of skills that make life as a medical student more tolerable. Most of these involve creating the impression that you know more than you actually do. This means avoiding answering questions about which you know nothing (which at the beginning is most things). Consider the ritual of bedside teaching. I made it my mission to avoid speaking to or touching the patients at all costs. Avoiding eye contact is a guaranteed way to be asked a question! All patients are examined from the right hand side, therefore initially it is advisable to stand on the left hand side of the patient. One needs to judge the time accurately, however, when the clinician will try to be cunning and ask the student standing the *furthest away* from the patient. The skilled student will anticipate this moment and, at the appropriate time, enthusiastically stands on the right of the patient, hence double bluffing the clinician. When successful this manoeuvre is poetry in motion.

After clinic I went to the casualty department, as it was my turn to shadow the house officer on call. This turns out to be highly enjoyable; seeing real patients with real diseases and being involved in the process of sorting them out without the responsibility of having to *know* things or make decisions. In the space of a few hours we see two old ladies with chest infections, a man with heart failure, two paracetamol overdoses, and a heart attack. A moment's peace some 4 or 5 hours later is shattered by a series of piercing bleeps and a crackling disjointed voice proclaims from the house officer's pocket that there has been a cardiac arrest on one of the wards. The dreaded crash bleep: we get up, and we run. We arrive on the ward, and very quickly there is a small crowd of doctors and nurses around the bed of the old man we had admitted earlier with a heart attack. I stand back feeling more than a little useless. Intrigued and a little appalled, I watch as the registrar gives instructions to insert lines and tubes and to administer drugs and electric shocks. After about 20 minutes everything stops; a stillness replaces the activity and the old gentleman is left to rest in peace. I feel upset and shocked, but to everyone else it's just part of the job.

The clinical years are the first real opportunity to manage your own time. It is important to do so sensibly. The system is open to abuse and many a cunning student manages to do the minimum amount of work in the shortest period of time. There will be things you love about being a student and things you'll hate. I personally would avoid operating theatres like the plague. There is nothing pleasant about standing around in green pyjamas, a paper shower cap, and fetid, communal shoes in which most decent people would not even grow mushrooms, never mind put their feet. The student in theatre is meant to *retract*. This involves pulling very hard on metal implements (which are usually inserted in a stranger's abdomen) in directions that your body was not designed to go. This causes pain, stiffness, and eventually loss of sensation in the hands, the likes of which have never been felt before outside a Siberian salt mine. It is important to learn the things you need to get through the examinations, but there are a lot of other valuable lessons to learn. One day you will be a house officer and your social life and sanity will be seriously compromised … so don't waste the time you have now. Medicine *is* great, with something to appeal to everyone. It's a little like a pomegranate: you will hopefully find it satisfying and worth while in the end, but it can be challenging and infuriating going through the process!

MB

Self-directed learning plays an ever increasing part as time goes on through the course and as you will be repeatedly reminded "every patient is a learning opportunity". There are always patients to be clerked and examined. This may be in the holistic mould of learning about the person, their condition, and the whole experience of their illness or learning the clinical features and management of the diseases relating to the speciality you are currently studying. Students nearing their clinical finals adopt a rather more focused approach: racing around the wards examining "the massive liver in bed 4", "the wheezy chest in bed 9", and the "rather embarrassing rash in the sideward", grabbing a quick coffee while firing questions at each other about the causes of finger clubbing and the side effects of amiodarone, then fitting in a couple of children and a mad person before lunch.

Keen students who spend more time on the wards seeing patients and learning about conditions for themselves often benefit from impromptu, informal teaching from junior doctors who can teach during the course of completing their ward work. Following a junior doctor on call is very valuable experience and is often the best way to see a general mix of cases. Students need to be around when things happen if they are not only to learn but to experience the excitement and satisfaction of clinical medicine. A group of students once reported on their experience in these words:

Our teaching was really, really good from house officers right through to consultants. So much time and effort was put in for us at all hours of the night and day, so much so that some of us learnt some important skills like how to read electrocardiograms (ECGs) in the early hours of the morning on take in the hospital.

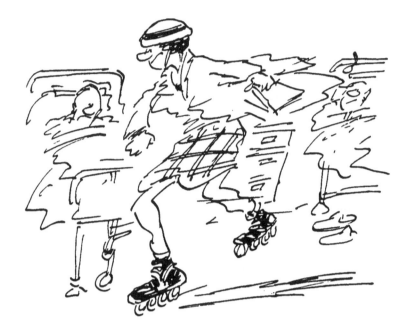

Spending an evening with the registrar in the accident and emergency department on the front line, seeing patients brought in by ambulance or referred by local GPs, is far more interesting for most students than standing at the back of an operating theatre, craning your neck, and still not being able to see what the surgeon is doing and getting flustered when you are shouted at for getting in the way or because you have momentarily forgotten the anatomical borders of Hasselback's triangle.

A night in casualty

I remember my first night in casualty as a medical student as one of the most exciting times of my whole medical training. My placement in what is properly called accident and emergency medicine was relatively early in my time at medical school so, although I felt that my knowledge was minimal, my enthusiasm levels had never been higher; how many other students would be excited at the prospect of spending all of Friday night doing college work? The department resembled Piccadilly Circus, in all senses, especially noise and smell. There was a constant flow of people milling here and rushing there, lying on trolleys, sitting on floors, banging on the wall, singing in the toilet, crying in the corner, or sleeping in the waiting room; men, women, children, patients, relatives, doctors, nurses, porters, receptionists, radiographers, a couple of burly policemen and a rather conspicuous and obvious plain clothed detective, and to cap it all two nuns looking for a missing mother superior.

As well as the large number of walking wounded, an increasing proportion of whom as the night wore on and the pubs closed became staggering wounded, there were a couple of cases which I think I will never forget as they showed me medicine in all its glory. A lovely lady in her 80s was brought in by ambulance, acutely short of breath and looking extremely distressed and scared. She had heart failure and her lungs were filling up with fluid as her heart could no longer pump effectively. Within minutes the junior doctor I was following around had put in a drip and was giving her some drugs which I had learnt about only a few weeks before in a tutorial. As I stood by her bed filling in the blood forms trying to help out a bit, she started to get her breath back and soon was able to talk to me. Within an hour she had managed to tell me her whole life story, including her several boyfriends during the war, the relevance of which to her medical history I still find hard to grasp, but she insisted it was important. About 2 a.m. a young man of my age was rushed in from a road traffic accident, having been knocked off his motorcycle at high speed. He was unconscious and had several broken bones. Seemingly out of nowhere an enormous group of doctors and nurses appeared in the resuscitation room and pounced on the man, but with awe inspiring calm and organisation; it really was like watching an episode of *Casualty*, except that on television you get a better view than you do when you are right at the back of a group of frantically busy people and you are trying not to get in the way. By 3.30 a.m. everything had quietened down somewhat, though the waiting area was still half full. The motorcyclist was in theatre having one of his fractures screwed together, and the sweet old lady with an interesting history was apparently soundly asleep on a ward, one of the lucky few not having to stay on a trolley in casualty. I wandered off to bed exhausted and exhilarated; the doctors and nurses carried on seeing patients. How, I wondered, will I ever know what to do and be able to treat people as well as they did, and, more worrying, how will I be able to stay awake that long?

GR

One of the most valuable experiences towards the end of training, which most schools encourage, is a period of several weeks shadowing a junior doctor. This usually occurs in medicine, surgery, or obstetrics and may take place in a general hospital away from the medical school. This allows only one or two students to be placed in each location, maximising their exposure to patients and teaching, and giving the opportunity for close supervision as clinical skills such as bladder catheterisation or intravenous cannulation are practised.

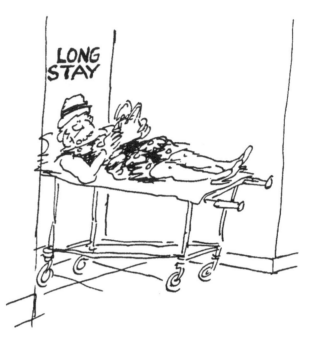

First delivery

I was woken up by the sound of my bleep. It was barely 4 a.m., and I had been asleep for less than 2 hours. By the time I had wearily put on my shoes and rushed to her cubicle, she had already begun to push. Jane, the midwife, decided that there was not time for me to put on a gown, so I just put on the gloves. The mother to be began to scream as the contractions became stronger and with each push the baby descended further. I placed my left hand on the head as the crown appeared to stop it rushing out too quickly, while supporting the mother with my right. I could almost feel my heart thumping against my chest. Any remaining signs of tiredness had now completely disappeared in all the excitement. Here I was minutes away from helping to bring a new life into the world.

It all went so quickly after that. First the baby's head appeared, and I pulled it down gently to release the anterior shoulder. The rest appeared to come out all by itself. It was 4.36 a.m. precisely, and a big baby boy was born. The mother cried with joy as I placed him on her tummy. It's an amazing feeling. The family wouldn't let me go until they had taken a photograph of me holding him in my arms. By the time I had helped the midwife clear the mess and made sure all was well, it was way past 5 a.m. Time to get some sleep.

FI

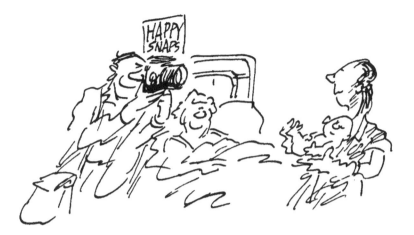

The clinical subjects

The major subjects to be learnt are general medicine and general surgery, and these are often studied in several blocks throughout the later years. Increasingly, the emphasis is on core clinical skills rather than an encyclopaedic knowledge of different disciplines. The boundaries between "subjects" are blurred and they are learned in a more integrated way and examined in integrated clinical examinations. If they are not integrated, and as medicine and surgery become ever more specialised, the best general experience is often achieved by rotating through several firms covering a range of subjects as well as being around when the firm is "on take" (the team responsible for general admissions on that day). An 8 weeks medical attachment may involve a fortnight each of chest medicine, infectious diseases, endocrinology, and cardiology. A similar rotation in surgery could include gastrointestinal surgery, vascular surgery, urology, and orthopaedics.

Generally, students are split into small groups and allocated to a particular firm in the relevant speciality. The firm is the working unit of hospital medicine and usually comprises a consultant or professor, one or two specialist registrars (who qualified several years before and are in training for that speciality), a senior house officer (who is usually a couple of years out of medical school and may be wanting to follow that speciality or may be in training for general practice or may just be drifting waiting for inspiration), and a house officer (who is newly qualified and will try and whisper the answers to the boss's questions to you, which is generally why you will get them wrong).

The patients in hospital (inpatients) under the care of that team also provide the teaching subjects for the students and are shared out between the students, who are expected to talk to their patients and examine them before being taught on ward rounds or teaching sessions by the senior members of the team. In the past much of this teaching was in the form of humiliation; ritualistic grillings of students in front of patient and colleagues alike, in the style of Richard Gordon's character Sir Lancelot Spratt and his blustering, "You boy! What's the bleeding time? Speak up. Speak up". While the occasional medical dinosaur can still be found eating a brace of medical students for lunch, it is no longer acceptable today and is much less likely to occur. The student who has taken the effort to prepare for such teaching can gain enormous benefit from seeing a condition he or she has previously only read about being illustrated in flesh and blood, making far easier the committing to memory of facts and figures as they suddenly take on real meaning and significance.

The use of community-based services as resources for learning is growing in all schools, some at a faster rate than others. For example, Bristol now has a series of clinical academies across the West Country in Bath, Swindon, and Taunton for instance, where students spend several months at a time on attachment to various teaching firms. As more care passes from hospital to community, such as in mental illness or child health, and as hospital stays tend to be much shorter, such as after having a baby or having day surgery, students are having to go to where the patients are.

GPs are playing an increasing part in undergraduate teaching of clinical skills, such as examination of body systems, in addition to their traditional role of teaching consultation skills and health promotion. Insight can also be gained into a broader spectrum of disease and social problems than is apparent in hospitals, learning to deal appropriately with minor everyday illnesses or major personal upheavals that affect people's lives.

A day in general practice

My practice starts the day with a team meeting. A coffee fix gives everyone time to label the important events of the next few days. The builders are in, so all hearts will have a continuous murmur today; a new software package will be demonstrated to allow current problems to be highlighted while listing previous diagnoses, but will it really help?

Instantly I am involved, my opinion sought in a warm welcome to the group. I ask what book I should read to learn about general practice and am told *Middlemarch* by George Eliot. Six months later, having read the book, I am still thinking about what was meant by that answer. In return, they ask me what skills a doctor should have in general practice. Everyone joins in, and the discussion leads us into seeing the patients.

Today I see the patients on my own first. I receive more trust and responsibility from these doctors in a week than in a year at the hospital. Presenting the complaint and my thoughts to the GP is excellent practice at developing a "problem-oriented approach". I am daunted by the impossibility of knowing the person and their history in 10 minutes, and hospital clerkings are little preparation. The long relationship between GP and patient is such a privilege and opportunity for appropriate intervention relevant to the patient's needs and wishes.

I think through the messages I learnt from watching myself on video being "consulted" by actors back at the St Mary's department of general practice. The skills are those of good listening, while considering the possible background to the presenting problem – the family problems, alcoholism – and the needs, articulated or unspoken, for caring, a further specialist opinion, or a prescription. I remember the advice that a holistic viewpoint and the availability of complementary therapies can obviate the need for drugs as psychological props for either doctor or patient.

Mr A has low back pain and was given short shrift by the orthopaedic consultant for not having sciatica that would be worth operating on, entirely ignoring his pain. We talk about his weight, posture, and stress at work and re-emphasise his need for exercises and a good chair, which seems more appropriate. Ms B comes in with severe abdominal pain and iliac fossa pain and rebound tenderness. My excitement at a possible hospital referral dies down as the doctor reassures both of us that this is constipation.

The case mix is so different in a teaching hospital; a sense of proportion is vital and can come only with experience. Mr C was found to be hypertensive opportunistically at a previous visit, and the nurse has confirmed this subsequently. We discuss what this implies for his future health and treatment, and the doctor and I talk afterwards about current concepts in the management of blood pressure from both personal care and population health perspectives. Every person is different and requires integrating and understanding of the possible pathologies with what is realistic in their life. Without time or fast investigations nearly every diagnosis may be provisional; "come back tomorrow" is not a cop-out but good management.

In the corridor we have a "kerbside" case conference about what to do with Ms X. She has many problems, and all the partners have been to visit her at one time or other. The latest news is not good, and, although she has heart failure, it is her mobility and risk of hip fracture that we worry about. We visit her before lunch, assess her cardiovascular and neurological status, and find out how well the carers are coping. It may be that improving the lighting will counter her drowsiness and prevent a disastrous fall.

Over lunch we discuss strategies and priorities in looking after someone with diabetes and the implications for GPs of the new National Health Service (NHS) changes. The balance has swung away from clinical freedom; doctors have lost much control over their time and decisions but to quite an extent are being forced to do what they would have liked to do anyway, namely more work on prevention and health promotion. Computerisation has been unavoidable but as yet wastes far more time than it saves. There is great potential for clear presentation of patient information and for networking outcomes between patients and practices for audit and research. I sit in quietly as another partner runs a yoga class in her lunchbreak and feel greatly refreshed for the afternoon.

Later on, I join the local community psychiatric nurse. One of the people we visit has panic attacks when she goes outside. The nurse has given her mental exercises to do at home and a routine to use when she feels the panic attack developing. We take her out for a walk calmly and get along without her anxiety becoming panic, which encourages her greatly. Another woman has gradually become more depressed since her husband died, and the nurse is delighted that she has a chance to intervene with counselling and cognitive therapy before a doctor (not from my practice!) has filled her full of tricyclic antidepressants. A third has Alzheimer's disease, and the issue is whether she will leave the frying pan on and burn the house down while her son is out at work.

Back at the practice I get on my bike to go home, overwhelmed by the breadth of insight needed in this work. The loneliness in the consulting room is more than compensated by the warmth of genuine teamwork and equal exchange of views and approaches. Humanity and pathophysiology do mix after all.

TA

The major clinical subjects in addition to medicine and surgery are also taught in a similar fashion: obstetrics (the care of pregnant women) and gynaecology (the speciality devoted to diseases confined to women); paediatrics (child health); and psychiatry (the care of patients with mental illness).

Other specialities occupy a smaller part of the students' time, and only a general understanding is required as detailed knowledge is beyond the scope of basic general medical training. These include neurology (disorders of the motor and sensory function of the brain, spinal cord, and peripheral nerves); rheumatology (medical disorders of joints such as arthritis); genitourinary

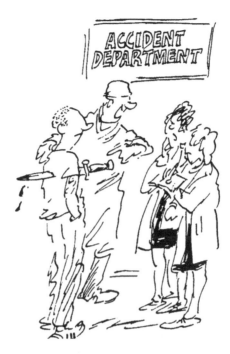

medicine (sexually transmitted diseases which may involve the study and care of human immunodeficiency virus (HIV) and acquired immunodeficiency syndrome (AIDS)); dermatology (skin diseases); ophthalmology (eye diseases); ear, nose, and throat surgery; and anaesthetics, which also covers pain management.

An attachment in the accident and emergency department is one of the most popular parts of the course for most students. The glamorous image portrayed by television series is never all it is cracked up to be, but the excitement level is generally high, especially when there is the chance to be a useful pair of hands, suturing a laceration, helping the nurse put a plaster cast on the broken arm of a wriggling 5 year old, or providing chest compressions during a resuscitation.

At some stage in the later years a more detailed approach to pathology is required, and this may take the form of a block of lectures, tutorials, and practicals or may be covered throughout the later years alongside the relevant clinical attachments. The subjects studied under the heading of pathology are chemical pathology (the biochemical basis of diseases); histopathology (the macro and microscopic structure of diseased tissues);

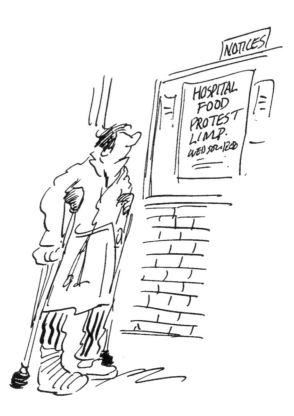

haematology (the diseases affecting blood and bone marrow); microbiology (combining the study of bacteria, viruses, and other infectious organisms); and immunology (the role of the immune system in disease). Without a knowledge of these disease processes it is difficult to understand clinical signs and symptoms and to interpret the results of laboratory tests which play a crucial part in diagnosis and management of patients.

Other topics are fitted in as the course progresses including clinical pharmacology and therapeutics (the prescribing of drugs to treat illness), palliative medicine (the care of the dying), medical law and ethics, more advanced communication skills such as breaking bad news and bereavement counselling, and sometimes personal care (how to look after yourself with all the physical and emotional stresses and strains of being a doctor) and basic management skills. An increasing number of medical schools also give students a general introduction to complementary and alternative medicine, so that as doctors they may have at least some insight into their patients' choices and also consider whether some aspects, such as acupuncture, might become a useful adjunct to their own practice. The aim of the later years is to build on the basic knowledge and skills learnt in the early years and to add to that the necessary attitudes and skills in decision making, coping with uncertainty, and dealing effectively with patients, relatives, and colleagues that patients should expect of a good doctor.

The elective

As well as the special study modules which allow each student choices in the precise content of their course, and the opportunity to learn how to study in greater depth, all schools set time aside in the later years of the course for what is known as the elective period. This is usually between 6 and 12 weeks long and is an opportunity for a student to undertake any medically related study at home or abroad. Most students take the chance to travel and see medicine being practised in a very different setting whether in a trauma unit in down town Washington DC, the Australian Flying Doctor Service, or a children's immunisation clinic in a canoe in Sarawak. Some students carry out research while on elective or gain experience of a subject to which they have only limited exposure in their undergraduate course such as learning difficulties or tropical diseases. The *British Medical Journal* offers a different sort of opportunity through the Clegg scholarship for electives working in medical journalism. The excerpts that follow show just how diverse the choice of elective can be.

A "local" elective – Newcastle

My elective was based at a NHS GP practice in Newcastle, which has good professional relationships with various complementary therapists in the local area. I was given the opportunity to visit each of the therapists and obtained practical experience of the use of a number of complementary therapies including Traditional Chinese Medicine and Acupuncture, Herbal Medicine, Homeopathy, Naturopathy, Aromatherapy, Chiropractic, Osteopathy, Yoga, Tai-Chi, Reflexology, Hypnotherapy, Shiatsu, Biofeedback, Spiritual Healing, Bi-Aura Therapy, Magnetic Therapy and Crystal Therapy. I was able to meet patients who had experienced various therapies and obtain their perspectives on whether a particular treatment had proved to be beneficial for them.

A typical day during my elective involved spending the morning sitting in with a GP during surgeries to understand how complementary therapies can be integrated into primary care. I noticed that the GP took a holistic approach to medicine, focusing on the whole person and not just their symptoms. He has adopted various strategies to promote health and prevent disease such as ensuring all his asthma patients have peak flow meters and lending out blood pressure monitors to patients. He prescribed some herbal remedies and nutritional supplements such as isphagula husk for constipation. The surgery session was followed by a seminar on the concept of adopting a holistic approach to health and disease. These seminars covered a variety of topics including nutrition, music therapy, energy medicine, the use of complementary therapies in cancer care, and Ayurvedic medicine. After the seminar, I would spend the rest of the day with one of the therapists, for example a Homeopath. I was able to spend time with two homeopaths in Newcastle observing them with patients and talking to patients about their experiences with homeopathy. The homeopaths took a detailed history from their patients including their current problems, past medical history, current medication and diet and lifestyle choices. They focussed on gaining an understanding of the whole person. The patients were then prescribed homeopathic remedies designed to help relieve their symptoms. The homeopaths said that they had a lot of success treating children with skin conditions such as eczema, acne and psoriasis. The patients I met said that they generally felt better after their treatment. However, there is little scientific evidence to show that homeopathic medicines are effective, largely due to the fact that there have been relatively few high quality clinical trials. Many critics of homeopathy argue that its effectiveness in treating individual patients is largely due to the placebo effect, but the homeopaths counter this with the fact that homeopathic treatment has been shown to be effective in animals.

On completion of my elective, I feel that I have a greater understanding of the potential uses of complementary therapies, the procedures involved, and the associated benefits and risks. I hope this will make me better prepared to support patients who are using or who are interested in using complementary and alternative medicine.

LH

An elective abroad – Kilimatinde Hospital, Great Rift Valley, Tanzania

Although I had a wonderfully interesting elective, which opened my eyes to a remote part of the world I didn't know existed, my first time on the ward was pretty unpleasant. It smelt like a farm. I later found that this was because the hospital cows were kept next door. I also saw a rat on the ward round and couldn't help draw parallels between rats in Tanzania and the constantly reported MRSA in the UK. Although I went into theatre on a few occasions I did not assist as I assessed the HIV risk to be too high. I was amazed to see that the only intra-operative observations were heart rate and manual blood pressure readings every five minutes.

The dedicated staff at the hospital worked tremendously hard with amazing commitment and went to great lengths to not only teach us but also to learn from us. One of the best moments in this respect was when a lady with angina came to OPD. I taught them how we would treat it but the concept of life long medication is totally alien there and we ended up prescribing aspirin for a month and propranolol for a week. I hoped that, if we proved it would work, the patient would be willing to pay for long term medication. One of the doctors later bumped into her in the village and she was apparently amazed that all her symptoms had gone in a day!

My worst time at the hospital came ten days into my stay when I was confronted with a dead baby who had been brought by her parents with an infected umbilical cord after a home birth. As the baby was unwrapped from her mothers back I found myself hesitating about the "diagnosis". It was highly unnerving to observe the almost blasé attitude of the staff, but I later concluded that this was a solid sense of reality; also perhaps a survival mechanism. In three years of medicine in the UK I had never seen a youngster die. After just three weeks in Tanzania I had seen four. The mother carried the baby home for burial and I realised how time and energy consuming grief is in the UK, compared to here.

Severe burns were another common problem in the hospital. This was unsurprising as most people cooked on open fires in otherwise poorly lit rooms. These burns were simply treated with some pain relief and Vaseline gauze. One particularly memorable case was that of Edward who, despite having sustained third degree burns and possible inhalation injury, made a fantastic recovery. By the end of our elective he was a far happier boy than when we arrived and would roar with laughter when I, the "mzungu", tickled his uninjured left arm. A mzungu is a "white European traveller" and although not wholly courteous it is far better than the Maasai word: The Maasai christened travellers iloridaa enjekat – "those who confine their farts".

DRC

Assessments and examinations

Schools adopt different systems of assessing students' clinical progress. Most combine end of attachment assessments with a final Bachelor of Medicine (MB) examination at the end of the course, which were traditionally taken in one grand slam but are increasingly now divided up into different parts over a year or longer. The final MB consists of different sections in pathology,

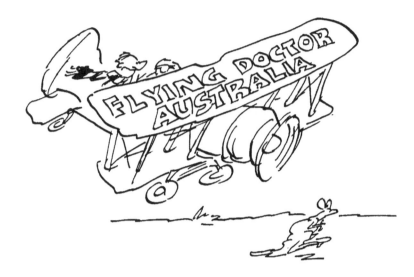

medicine, surgery, clinical pharmacology and therapeutics, and obstetrics and gynaecology. The "minor" speciality attachments are included in the major subjects. The amount of emphasis placed on each varies, and within each the emphasis is on the ability to reason and use knowledge rather than to function as a mixture between a sponge and a parrot. Some schools prefer almost total continuous assessment with each examination contributing to the final MB. Others continue to put major emphasis on finals with the regular assessments being used to monitor progress and certify satisfactory attendance and completion of an attachment.

An increasing number of schools split finals into two, with the written papers taken a year earlier than clinicals, to encourage concentration on clinical skills and decision making before becoming a house officer. The final MB comprises multiple choice questions, extended answers to structured questions, or essays, and practicals. In medicine (which includes paediatrics and psychiatry), surgery, and obstetrics and gynaecology considerable emphasis is placed on the clinical bedside examination, which tests skills in talking to patients, eliciting the relevant clinical signs, and making a diagnosis. Oral examinations are also held in most subjects. Clinical skills are increasingly being tested in a more systematic way through Objective Structured Clinical Examinations (OSCEs). A few minutes are spent by all candidates at a series of "stations" at which they have to perform a particular task, or address a problem.

However the examinations are structured, there is no avoiding the fact that they require considerable amounts of work over a prolonged period. They are as much a test of emotional stability and physical endurance as they are of knowledge and skills. Most students do pass at their first attempt; up to 10% have to resit all or part of their finals 6 months later. Very few fail more than once.

REMEMBER

- The later years are more like being an apprentice than a conventional student.

- The course is largely concerned with core clinical skills, strategies of investigation and treatment, and professional attitudes.

- Much of the learning is from patients, including acute emergencies, and at times it is necessary for students to live in the hospital overnight or occasionally for longer periods.

- Students may travel to nearby hospitals, community health centres and GP surgeries for a broader exposure to medical practice.

- The main clinical components are the principles and practice of general medicine and surgery and their related subspecialities: obstetrics and gynaecology, child health, psychiatry, clinical pharmacology and therapeutics, and the underlying pathology sciences. Communication skills and ethics continue as important themes.

- Choice and opportunities for study in depth are provided through special study modules which may be expanded to lead to an intercalated science degree.

- The elective period, which most students spend abroad, is a great opportunity to travel and learn how medicine is practised in other countries and cultures.

- Assessment in the later years is by a mixture of in-course and end-of-course assessments and final examinations, testing clinical skills, attitudes, and ability to use the knowledge gained. The pattern of assessment used varies substantially between schools.

- Up to 10% of students may fail one or more parts of their finals on one occasion but most are successful at a second attempt.

9

Doubts

Doubts are a very normal part of most people's lives. No university course, and no professional training, is more likely to raise doubts than medicine: academic doubts, vocational doubts, and personal doubts.

As Richard Smith, formerly editor of the *British Medical Journal*, once wrote:

Once they arrive, medical students are put through a gruelling course and exposed younger than most of their non-medical friends to death, pain, sickness, and what the great doctor William Osler called the perplexity of the soul. And all this within an environment where "real doctors" get on with the job and only the weak weep or feel distressed. After qualification, doctors work absurdly hard, are encouraged to tackle horrible problems with inadequate support, and then face a lifetime of pretending that they have more powers than they actually do. And all this within an environment where narcotics and the means to kill yourself are readily available. No wonder some doctors develop serious problems.

Few would-be medical students never have reservations whether medicine is right for them and they for medicine. All too often these doubts have concentrated too much on the process of getting into medical school and too little on what being a doctor is all about, the consequence of which being to add to the cynicism and disillusionment which is rife among junior doctors. After working for several years on the BBC television series *Doctors To Be*, the producer Susan Spindler recognised this problem and offered some good advice:

It's hard to take a career decision at the age of 17; at that age many people haven't quite decided who they are and many of us change almost beyond recognition between the ages of 17 and 25. If you are in any doubt about your suitability for the medical life, postpone the decision: do another degree first and wait until you are certain before entering medicine. Even if you've been set on becoming a doctor since you were a young child, do

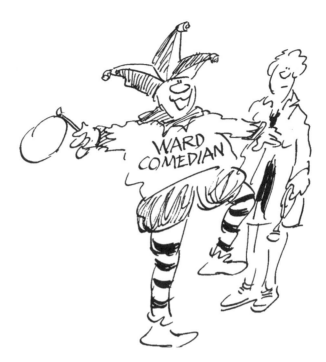

your homework first: spend time with as many doctors as you can – in hospitals and surgeries, doing different kinds of jobs. Get a clear idea of the range of possibilities that medicine can offer.

Once at medical school not many students survive 5 years without wondering if they are on the right track. Doctors in the early years after qualification are almost universally nagged with doubts about finding jobs, obtaining higher qualifications, and whether their aspirations are realistic in terms of skills and opportunities. With increasing numbers of medical graduates from UK medical schools and qualified doctors from across the European Union, the competition for training posts and senior medical jobs is becoming tougher than ever before. The cosy security of a job-for-life that many previous generations of doctors enjoyed is perhaps under threat as medicine is exposed to the harsh realities of commercialism and consumer demand that other professions have also seen.

Alongside these academic and vocational doubts the world of doctors in training also creaks and groans with all the normal difficulties of men and women finding their feet in an adult world. If newly away from home they must find accommodation and adjust to the responsibilities that brings. Mature students must acclimatise to a world that is often very different, more hierarchical, and sometimes also more juvenile than that in which their feet have been so firmly planted for some years. Coping with the financial difficulties, experienced by most students but particularly self-funding mature students, can take its toll. Medical students are not immune to all the usual identity crises that strike most other students at some stage nor the relationship dramas. In some ways the pressure to conform that pervades medicine in general, and in medical schools in particular, does nothing to make such problems easier; the pressure on time, especially at examination times and in the early years after qualification, can test even the strongest of personal involvements.

Academic doubts

Academic doubts at medical school are common in the early years. As the first set of examinations or assessments approaches, most students feel nervous about the amount of work they should be undertaking. The subject matter and the style of learning and of examinations may be very different from previous experience. The greater emphasis on self-directed learning with less of the spoon feeding by teachers that many students are used to from school can be bewildering at first. It is also much more difficult initially to gauge the amount of work to do from seeing other people working. As at school there will always seem to be individuals, who sail through examinations with apparent ease on minimal revision, while you spend months solidly slaving away just to scrape a pass. You will also soon find out the weird and wonderful ways some of your new friends have of studying. Some will stay up all night, others will have done 4 hours' work before breakfast, some seem to stay up all day and all night, while one of your flatmates will still seem to be going to hockey practice, then for a drink with friends, then coming home for an early night. Of course, only the very exceptional cases do as little work as they seem to, and the best way to dispel any doubts as to how much work to do is to do as much as you can; the vast majority of people who fail examinations at medical school do so because they do too little too late. You should remember that you have already proved with your entrance requirements that you are academically capable of getting through the course, provided you apply yourself realistically to the task ahead.

Vocational doubts

Doubts of a very different nature often surface when you are faced with dealing with patients. Often this is because of the perception of the student that their need to learn from the patient without really contributing directly to their management makes them feel they are intruding and that the patient is resentful of their involvement. This is rarely the case, and a student with more time to spend talking than busy junior doctors can make a considerable contribution to the care of patients, most of whom also fully recognise that we all have to learn somewhere and on someone. One patient described her experience like this.

My student

There must come a time when books and lectures need to be supplemented with real experience on real patients. Most people are happy to oblige; after all they are altruistic enough to give blood and carry organ donor cards, and it is more agreeable to give students access to your live body than to donate it for "spare parts".

I was first examined by students during one of my pregnancies. I had to rest in hospital for several weeks and was captive for any passing student to listen to my heart murmur and my baby's heart: two for the price of one.

Recently I was in hospital again. The relationship between student and patient can be mutually beneficial. The student can be a comforting presence, having more time to spend with the patient than the busy registrar on his or her brisk ward round, and the student's attention is a welcome break in the crushing boredom of life in a hospital ward. Do not underestimate the importance of a student's interest in a patient. Other patients watch enviously as the curtains are swished closed round your bed, ears strain to hear what is going on inside.

My student last time was a girl and quite young. She was extremely polite, with a warm friendly approach, which helped me to relax. My permission was sought and I agreed to let her examine me, literally from head to toe. I touched my nose; my eyes followed her pen as she moved it across my visual field; I wriggled my toes for her, I must confess to a feeling of slight amusement as she consulted her highlighted textbook as we completed each test. She even admitted that it was the first time she had done this. I was quite touched.

My student had to take my medical history and present it to the rest of the team. She seemed to be very thorough, much more thorough than an earlier student in her final year. She was relaxed and spoke confidently about my case and having done

> her homework answered all the questions that were fired at her. I felt she did well and that she already has a good bedside manner.
>
> Occasionally it is possible to recognise a former student after they have qualified. I was visiting a patient in hospital when this happened. The doctor came to see the patient, and as she turned to go she actually remembered me; I was so pleased. I could not help noticing that gone was her slightly hesitant student manner, apologising for having cold hands; in its place was a brisk confident doctor doing a great job in a busy hospital. How proud I felt to have played a small part.

Learning from patients, especially in the early years, can occasionally be disturbing and unsettling. Coming to terms with blood, disfigurement, suffering, disability, mental illness, incurable disease, and death is difficult for all students, but most will overcome it without becoming hard and completely detached. A few others find it hard to relate to patients, which is then compounded by them failing to develop the essential skills in talking to and examining patients. Usually the best remedy in these cases is to engineer a greater degree of involvement and responsibility, but with more and better communication skills teaching in schools now such students can find a good deal of help available. Occasionally this gulf seems unbridgeable, and the student may have to decide whether to change course or to press on to qualification in the knowledge that many career options in medicine have limited contact with patients.

Personal doubts

The number of young doctors leaving medicine is nothing like as high as has been reported. Fewer than 5% change career in the first 5 years after qualification. Any loss at this stage represents a substantial waste of public money; but, more than that, any waste of bright, talented, motivated, dedicated individuals with ideals and aspirations which led them to become doctors in the first place and who, for whatever reasons, decide to give up is a tragedy. The factors which lead to disillusionment in young doctors are numerous (even if they do not leave medicine), often resulting from a feeling that their expectations and aspirations are being thwarted – whether by failing postgraduate exams or not securing the desired training post or because the demands of the job can simply be tough at times. Some of the problem, however, lies with the junior doctors themselves. Too many doctors admit they did not know what they were letting themselves in for. Nor perhaps did they realise the limitations of medicine to meet the high expectations of the public – or of themselves. The earlier the problem is examined the better: perhaps the combination of an improvement in working conditions and a generation of enlightened, well-informed new doctors with an understanding of what lies ahead will lead to better morale and less waste.

Given the breadth of talent of most successful applicants to medical school it should come as little surprise that a major concern for many doctors is that they have "sold their soul to medicine" and are now incapable of doing anything else. In reality, many simply feel trapped in a job they begin to resent. They feel they have lost, or had knocked out of them, all the dreams and potential they had when they arrived at medical school. An old Chinese aphorism states: "You grow old not by having birthdays, but by deserting ideals", and being a tired, harassed, stressed junior doctor makes you feel prematurely old. Perhaps there is much that can be done within the structure of medicine to prevent "burn out" but doctors sometimes need reminding that "the grass is always greener ...". There is no escaping the

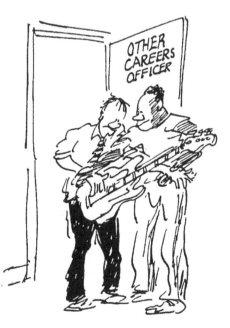

fact that medicine is not just a job but also a way of life. It is important to realise that far from being less likely than others to have serious problems, doctors are in some ways more likely to. They need to be prepared to discuss their problems and to seek appropriate help. Susan Spindler, producer of the *Doctors To Be* series, had this to say about doubts and some ways of dealing with them:

The early years as a qualified doctor can be so tough that they test the strongest of vocations. A supportive network of family and friends – people on whom you can offload anxieties and with whom you can share traumatic experiences – can make the difference between staying and quitting. You need all the student qualities listed above [see pp. 28–30] plus initiative and the ability to take decisions. A robust value system that isn't driven by the pursuit of riches – you'll probably see school and university peers working far shorter hours for far more money during your late 20s and early 30s. A need to compromise on the wish to achieve all you can in your career *and* forge a relationship/marriage and raise a family – a particular source of difficulty for women in hospital medicine. A supportive partner or spouse certainly makes life much easier. And, if you have managed to keep a circle of non-medical friends, you'll reap the rewards now: many doctors find themselves trapped in a world of medical politics and socialising – it's much easier to maintain a balanced view of life if some of the people you spend time with are not doctors.

Vocational doubts and academic failures occasionally occur during the course because of psychiatric illness, which is sometimes the outcome of relentless parental pressure to follow a career which a student either did not want or for which he or she was unsuited. Depression is the usual response. Expert advice is needed. Psychiatric illness may be self-limiting but it may be persistent or recurrent and incompatible with the standards of service and judgement which patients have a right to expect.

The importance of seeking help and advice before problems become overwhelming cannot be too strongly emphasised. Most difficulties tend to grow if incubated. In the first place there is no substitute for sharing problems with good friends, and that is one reason why a successful school needs to be a happy, considerate community and not just an academic factory. But the advice of friends may need to be supplemented by tutors, other teachers, and doctors in the students' health service, pastors, priests, or parents. Although it is true that a problem shared is a problem halved, a problem anticipated can be a problem avoided. No problems are unique and none insuperable.

Very occasionally the right move is to change course, in which case the sooner the better. To change direction for good reason is the beginning of a new opportunity, not a disaster.

One thing is reasonably certain: decisions either to learn medicine or to abandon the task should not be taken too quickly. As Lilian Hellman wrote in *The Little Foxes*: "Sometimes it's better to let the sun rise again".

REMEMBER

- Doubts are a normal part of everyone's life.

- Most doubts are about personal ability and career aspirations.

- Mature students, more than most, have moments when they question whether they are doing the right thing.

- Anyone who has achieved the entry requirements to medical school need have no doubts about academic ability. Academic failure normally only results from working too little, too late, and in a disorganised way.

- The few who will have doubts about relating to patients can be helped through communication skills training.

- Unrealistic expectations can lead to doubts but can be avoided, and prevention lies in an honest appraisal of oneself and careful researching before opting for the career.

- Occasionally, the decision to enter medicine turns out to be a mistake. Changing course or career is a brave move, which can lead to a new and more fulfilling life.

- The best remedy for doubts is to share them with someone; you will find you are not alone.

10

The new doctor

Almost all medical students would agree that the final examinations for their medical degree, whatever form they take, are the most terrifying and daunting experience of their lives. That is until a few weeks later when they walk onto the wards for the first time as a "proper doctor". After 4 to 6 years preparing for this day, you are thrust headlong into the real world. To become a really proper doctor, that is to be a fully registered medical practitioner, the General Medical Council (GMC) requires each new doctor to complete a year of satisfactory service in an appropriately supervised, educationally supported pre-registration house officer post. This is the first year of the 2-year Foundation Programme which begins the postgraduate training phase of the doctor's career. Major reforms of medical training and the application processes have been in put in place in recent years and, as in so many aspects of healthcare, continued reform is promised. The intention is to give a broader base of experience in a variety of specialities. It is thus argued that a more informed choice can be made as to which speciality one may choose after the Foundation Programme and that is produces a more 'well-rounded' doctor. While the aims of many of these reforms are laudable in terms of ending the influence of the "old-boy network" on job applications and making the systems more streamlined, transparent and fairer, in reality the wholesale introduction of an electronic centralised system has had significant teething troubles which have made a stressful time in a doctor's life even more uncertain.

The real world

In a white coat, never again to be so clean and tidy, with pockets bulging with books, pens, notepads, and all manner of equipment you have little idea how to use, you walk proudly onto the ward to be met by a roll of the eyes ("Oh God, it's August again!") from the formidable ward sister. A couple of hours later your sparkle of youthful enthusiasm has transformed into a downcast look of dread and horror. You have been introduced, albeit fleetingly, to your team, and one of them actually said hello. Or at least that is what you assume he meant when he grunted at you from behind a huge pile of patient files in the tiny, windowless doctors' office.

Now for the patients. There are quite a few of them at the moment because the team was "on take" at the weekend and the old infirmary up the road has been closed down and is being turned into luxury flats. You frantically try to write down everything your predecessor is telling you even though most of it makes no sense to you. There is no time to ask questions because her next job is in the Shetland Islands and she was due to start 3 hours ago. Then your bleep goes off: a patient needs to be admitted from the emergency department and his relative is complaining that he has been waiting for half an hour already and he's going to write to his MP. Then you have to go for a computer induction course but you can't find where it is. You also need the toilet but you can't find that either. And your consultant's secretary has just called you and asked you to take some notes to your boss in clinic. On the way you stumble across a scruffy looking elderly gent slumped in the corner of the lift. Is he drunk or just asleep? You are fairly sure he is breathing, but just in case you get out at the next floor and use the stairs. Your bleep goes again: Mrs Smith needs some paracetamol but you can't remember the dose; Mr Jones needs a new drip siting, and you always missed on the model as a student but this time it's for real; and Mr Patel's son has just arrived and wants to know the latest about his father's test results, and you remember it was bad news. There is still that patient in accident and emergency (A&E) and the consultant now needs an X-ray, which is in the boot of his BMW.

It's now 4 o'clock in the afternoon, no lunch yet, and come to think of it, you still haven't found a toilet. Your registrar is now waiting on the ward to go round all the patients to check you've done all the jobs from this morning.

Suddenly after 6 years in the sanctuary of the medical school, this is the real world of the house officer. All the older doctors will keep telling you that you young 'uns don't know you're born these days and how they worked so much harder in their day.

The Foundation Programme

For those students (by far the majority) who pass their final examinations in June or July, a well-deserved summer holiday usually beckons before that fateful day in early August when they wake up one morning and go to the hospital, not as a mere medical student but as a new doctor.

The first part of the medical career is called the Foundation Programme. This consists of 2 years of supervised clinical work in specially designed posts enhanced by an integrated educational programme. During Foundation Year One (F1), the new doctor is a pre-registration house officer who has been given provisional registration by the GMC, the medical equivalent of "L-plates". Unless there are exceptional circumstances, these two years follow immediately after graduating and it is generally accepted that it is better for everyone to get them over and done with while all you have learned is fresh in your mind. Foundation Schools have been set up to manage the recruitment to the clinical jobs and oversee the educational programme, which supports those jobs. A national curriculum is now in place to ensure that, by the end of the Foundation Programme, each new doctor will have achieved the same generic clinical and non-clinical competences, regardless of the precise nature of the placements over the 2 years.

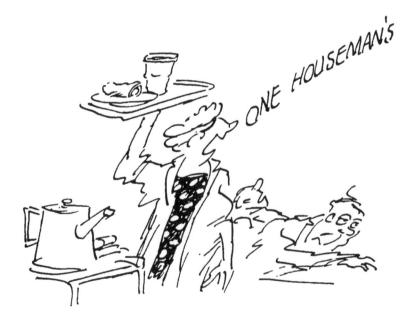

The F1 year will be spent in a series of three 4-month long rotating posts within the same or neighbouring hospitals. These will take the new doctor through some of the important general areas of required experience, such as general internal medicine and general surgery, as well as opportunities for exposure to more specialised areas. An example of a typical Foundation Year 1 rotation would be 4 months in General Medicine, 4 months of General Surgery and 4 months of General Practice. The second Foundation year could consist of 4 month rotations between Intensive Care, Orthopaedics and Public Health The new doctor will be expected to work with teams caring for both acute medical cases presenting to the hospital's emergency department as well as time spent caring for inpatients during their stays on the wards.

During the F1 year the new doctor will be expected to develop and demonstrate the core competencies of being a doctor – such as recognition and management of acutely unwell patients, practical clinical skills such as suturing wounds and inserting tubes into veins, and professional skills such as good record keeping, team working, and consultation skills. An educational supervisor will be appointed to guide each new doctor through this process, and assessing at the end of each post how much progress is being made and giving assistance where needed. At the end of this first year of work when the necessary competencies have been reached, the new doctor will acquire full registration from the GMC. They can then proceed to the second foundation year (F2), as a senior house officer, which will further develop their clinical training, prior to any move towards a choice of specialty.

Being a house officer

The house officer (or F1 doctor, a much less elegant term!) is the bottom rung of the medical ladder; it is no less important for that. The house officers spend much of their day on the wards providing the regular, front-line contact between the patients and the team of doctors looking after them. Much time is spent talking to new patients about the details of their illness or injury, examining them, ordering the initial investigations, and collating the results. In addition the house officer will often be responsible for documenting in the patients' notes the clinical decisions which the team has

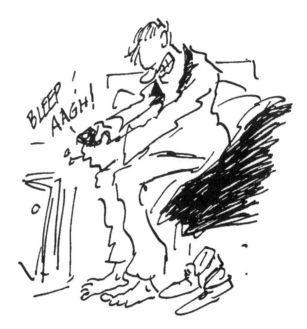

made about their management, and for enacting those decisions where possible. Much time is spent preparing the patient for the next step in their care, whether it is going to the operating theatre or getting ready to go home later that day. It is usually the house officer who is called when a patient needs pain control, or their fluid requirements need managing, or their discharge arrangements need to be sorted. Similarly those house officers who are attached to a clinical team delivering acute care to new arrivals at the emergency department, and increasingly in Admissions or Assessment Units, perform a similar role but with less continuity of care as patients are moved as quickly as possible to appropriate ward based teams. This speedier throughput of patients, is of course a good thing if you find yourself being a patient, but it does sometimes mean that the new doctor no longer has the opportunity of regularly seeing patients through the whole of their journey into hospital and then home again.

The house officer's role requires excellent communication skills involving as it does frequent face-to-face contact with patients and their relatives. Medical schools increasingly emphasise the development of such skills in students but no amount of practice sessions with actors simulating patients can fully prepare the new doctor for this most difficult of tasks. Many new doctors find the intimacy of the patient – doctor relationship exceptionally challenging, and most doctors (even the most experienced) would admit the challenge of dealing close up with pain, suffering, and the whole gamut of human emotions may diminish but never disappears. Like all the greatest challenges though, it also offers some of the most special rewards, like the patient with terminal cancer who, the night before she died, told her house officer that his care and kindness made her illness less terrifying and lonely than she had feared.

A status symbol

Being a junior doctor is not all the heart-wrenching stuff of television medical dramas. Neither is the job (for most people anyway) quite as filled with exciting action – both medical and romantic – as these television soaps would have us believe. One area that is rarely well portrayed is the central role played in the life of the house officer by the small black pager, which all junior doctors carry, called a bleep. It is one of the "status symbols" of a new doctor, largely because mere medical students are not regarded as sufficiently qualified to be given one.

After years as a student feeling a bit in the way on the wards, suddenly you are so important that if you are *not* there, you will be summoned to attend immediately by the shrill little noise of your bleep. It is a proud moment for all new (and *naïve*) doctors as they collect their bleep on their first day at work, and many head immediately for the nearest group of medical students to gloat and hope it goes off, just to illustrate their vital role in the healing of the sick. The novelty lasts almost until the end of the 2nd day, when most people have realised it is the albatross around their neck for the next decade.

One colleague's bleep number was the same four digits as the telephone extension of the hospital's Domestic Supervisor. It took her 3 weeks to realise that, as the Surgical house officer, the numerous calls she received were not actually meant for her and there was no need to keep running off to the Children's Ward with a mop and bucket to clean up more vomit. Another colleague was bleeped in the middle of the night to assess a patient who was shivering violently in his bed in a side room. Concerned he may have developed a dangerous fever, he raced from the comfort of his armchair in the doctors' mess to the ward. There he found a poor old soul lying on a bed with no blankets and next to a window that was wide open to the freezing December weather. "Six years at medical school just to close a bloody window" was the comment he was heard muttering under his breath as his stomped off back to his armchair. Some bleeps

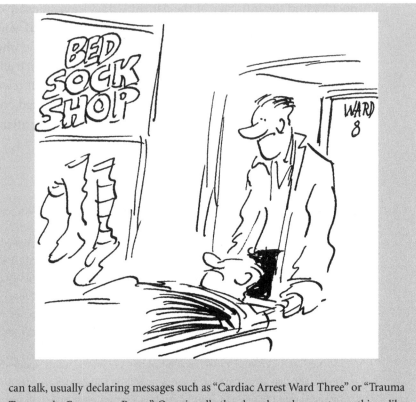

can talk, usually declaring messages such as "Cardiac Arrest Ward Three" or "Trauma Team to the Emergency Room". Occasionally they have been known to say things like "Fluid balance tutorial at 6 pm in the Floral-Regal Ethanol Unit" (which translates as "Anyone for beers after work in the Rose and Crown?"). As well as talking, these bleeps develop a mind of their own, and can therefore choose when to emit their, by now, detested screech. They know when you have just taken a bite of your sandwich at lunchtime, or when you are in the middle of explaining a colonoscopy to a hard of hearing elderly lady in a cubicle in A&E ("You want to put it where dear?"), or every time you attempt to go to the toilet.

Where to work

The Foundation Programme is designed to give more structured educational support to all new doctors, whatever post they are in. However, the clinical experience gained in different hospitals may vary greatly. Most prospective house officers look for jobs that best match their interests and career intentions, with most trying to obtain some balance and variety. Some students choose to undertake jobs in high profile teaching hospitals while others choose local district general hospitals. While each has its own pros and cons, achieving a good balance is also the aim of most Foundation Schools and candidates can expect to be placed in jobs throughout the two years in different types of hospital.

Work–life balance factors will also be taken into account: a keen surfer may well choose to be nearer the sea, while the dedicated night-clubber sticks to the urban jungle. Some new doctors have special ties to consider such as a spouse with or without children who cannot readily move to a new place. It is always worth talking to someone who has done the job recently that you think you want to do. They will be a mine of useful information about the reality of the job, rather than the hype. That will help you judge if the job would suit you and you would suit that job.

The hours

For many years, the high-spirited antics of medical students were forgiven by the public at large because as junior doctors they were sentenced to years of hard labour on meagre rations. It is certainly true that within the last 15 years, the working conditions for junior doctors have altered radically, partly from public and professional pressure and partly due to the influence of regulation from the European Commission. In many ways, these have been almost universally accepted as a good thing – with the occasional exception of the old-fart consultant who believed that only the weak-willed needed weekends off, or holidays, or sleep, or a decent salary. The main change came about in 1991 with a so-called "New Deal for Junior Doctors". This attempted to gradually reduce the total numbers of hours worked by junior doctors (which, in effect, meant anyone not a general practitioner (GP) or a consultant). Many doctors still in their mid-thirties can (and probably will) regale you of their 120 hour weeks as house officers (there are only 168 hours in a week) and of the infamous 3-day on-call weekends when they started work at 8 a.m. on Friday and left at 6 p.m. on Monday with no guarantee of any rest periods, sleep or even decent food.

The pace of change was speeded up however in 1998 when the British Government signed up to the European Working Time Directive. This health and safety measure is designed to protect the rights of workers across the European Union to acceptable conditions of employment to achieve a good work–life balance. In the field of health care, of course, there was the added benefit to the general public that the doctor taking out their appendix or delivering their baby at 3 a.m. might actually stay awake during the procedure.

Once implemented, the directive would be enforceable under law and the NHS could find itself in the European Court of Justice, facing huge fines (as well as political embarrassment) if it breached the strict new rules. The Government negotiated an exemption from this legislation for junior doctors until 1st August 2004, however since then all junior doctors' contracts have had to include:

- a maximum average number of hours worked of 58 per week (including on-call time)
- a daily continuous rest period of 11 hours
- a 20 minute rest break for each 6 hours worked in a shift
- a minimum of 24 hours continuous rest in each 7-day period or 48 hours in each fortnight
- a minimum of 4 weeks paid annual leave
- a maximum of 8 hours work in any 24 hours for night workers in stressful jobs

From 2009, the European Working Time Directive maximum working week for junior doctors will be 48 hours, so increasing the pressure on employers even further.

So, for the house officers of the future, there will be no more long hours, no more nights without sleep, or days without a meal. But also, as some have pointed out, no more sympathy from the general public and perhaps no more excuses for badly behaved medical students just "getting it out of their system, poor dears!".

More worryingly, many of the current leaders of the medical profession both young and old, have serious concerns that the vastly reduced hours may end up being counter-productive for patient care by reducing the overall clinical experience of doctors in training.

In addition to balancing the working conditions and training needs of junior doctors, the NHS also has the prime consideration of providing safe and effective clinical care to patients 24 hours a day. This balancing act is made even harder with the ever-increasing expectations of the public and the demands of politicians meaning more work to be done but less hours to do it in. The number of medical students has been increased and the numbers of medical graduates and therefore doctors in training is steadily increasing thereby sharing the workload. But doctors are having to adopt new ways of working. Hospitals up and down the country have tried numerous different ways of managing these competing priorities. Physicians' assistants are employed in some places to support medical teams with many of the less complicated but regular, routine tasks such as filling out forms and chasing test results. Nurses and therapists are expanding their roles taking on many clinical tasks previously regarded as the preserve of doctors, such as: prescribing of intravenous fluids and some medications; performing procedures such as endoscopies; running specialist outpatient clinics; admitting routine surgical patients to the ward; or dealing with minor ailments and injuries.

The biggest change, however, is the emergence of shift work replacing the traditional on-call rota. Increasingly the only way that adequate medical cover can be provided, within the limitations of junior doctors' new reduced hours, is to have in effect three doctors sharing a 24 hours period of cover in shifts. Within the last year or two a new doctor would have been expected to work five full days (9 a.m.–5 p.m.) and then at least one night per week staying at the hospital to cover the 5 p.m.–9 a.m. shift (perhaps with only a few hours of sleep interrupted with several calls to see a sick patient on the ward). Then the weekends and public holidays would be also covered in turn by say five or six house officers.

In previous years, only in the A&E Department did junior doctors undertake full shifts, like other jobs such as nurses or police officers. Now increasingly, full shifts are in operation. In many cases the intensity of work is more during these shifts, as less doctors are on call for the same numbers of patients. This could mean in an average week having three days working from 8 a.m.–4 p.m., then 2 days working 2 p.m.–10 p.m. The following week could then be a week of night shifts starting at 10 p.m. and finishing at 8 a.m. In addition, the continuity of care to patients may be reduced so doctors are required to undertake lengthy hand-over procedures when changing shifts to ensure the in-coming doctors are aware of all the current or possible medical complications that may occur in the next few hours with the patients entrusted to their care. A major drawback from a learning perspective is that you often never find out what happened to a particularly sick patient you dealt with previously; also the patient him/herself loses a familiar (hopefully friendly) face.

The pay

An outside observer may, however, be surprised to learn that some junior doctors are unenthusiastic about the new contracts. Despite some concerns over training and experience, it is true that in the last 10 years the hours worked has been cut in half while the salaries of new doctors have more than doubled, even taking account of inflation.

The pay of a junior doctor is calculated on the basis of a basic salary (approximately £22,000 per year gross in 2007/2008) topped up with a banding payment of between 20 and 80% of the basic. This banding payment depends upon:

• the number of hours worked exceeding 40 hours per week
• the intensity of the workload
• the amount of time spent working at antisocial hours

These bands are based on close monitoring of work diaries completed by junior-doctors. A foundation year house officer working in a post which is graded as Band 1a or 2b (the commonest bandings) will, for example, receive an additional 50% on top of the basic amount taking the total annual salary to approximately £32,000 a year. In addition to this you will be entitled to the highly regarded NHS Pension Scheme and your post may attract additional London Weighting payments.

Being a "Senior House Officer"

The second Foundation Year (F2) builds on the skills and competencies developed in the F1 year and the Senior House officer, as they are known, will usually pass seamlessly from their F1 year into a rotation of F2 posts within the same Foundation School. The focus for the curriculum in the F2 year is more on management of the acutely ill patient but continues to developed generic skills such as communication and team-working. At least one of the next placements is likely to be in a speciality which is currently under-doctored, another may be in general practice or a more unusual hospital speciality. This allows for graduates to experience a range of medical jobs perhaps giving them some exposure to something which interests them or at least allows them to see the profession from a colleague's perspective whatever their future career path. Some Foundation Schools also provide day-release taster schemes to allow for doctors to dip a toe in the water of a speciality they have never worked in but would like to see if only for the briefest of times.

It is also common immediately after this stage of your career to consider a period of time working abroad, and many opportunities exist, particularly in other English-speaking countries such as Australia, New Zealand, Canada, and South Africa whose medical systems and careers are broadly similar to the UK and where you can often work without the need to undertake further examinations (as you would need to do to work in the USA for example). Not too long ago, many young doctors feared being dismissed as "time-wasters" by future bosses if they spent say a year working in an A&E unit in Australia or as an expedition doctor in Africa but, increasingly, a more enlightened view exists and many consultants see working abroad as valuable experience in the juniors they employ.

The good life

Being a new doctor is not just about your first pay packet, however nice it is to see the beginning of the end to the debt-ridden years of medical school. The new doctor is uniquely placed to develop good patient–doctor relationships, to be involved in a team, putting 6 years of theory into practice, and not least having the feeling of doing a worthwhile job which still commands respect from the public. The hours may be shorter and the support more forthcoming, but being a new doctor is still tough work. It is emotionally demanding, and expectations are high from all concerned. At times like this, the friendships and camaraderie that typify medical students are worth their weight in gold.

There is a huge step up in terms of responsibility on becoming a Foundation Year doctor: the notorious medical student pub-crawls sometimes feel like light-years away, replaced by hectic ward rounds, endless discharge summaries and cardiac arrests. However, it is interesting to note that, while in the midst of facing the challenges of their first few years as a doctor, many see them as a means to an end, to be endured not enjoyed. Once it is over, however, and the doctor has stepped further up the career ladder, a surprising number of them look back on being a house officer and SHO as being some of the happiest days (and nights) of their lives.

REMEMBER

- After passing finals and graduating in medicine all new doctors commence a 2-year Foundation Programme, the 1st year of which is spent as a junior house officer and the 2nd as a senior house officer equivalent.

- Your medical degree qualifies you for provisional registration with the GMC. Successful completion of your first year entitles you to full registration.

- Junior doctors no longer work on average longer than 56 hours per week. In future this will reduce even further to 48 hours per week. This means that new doctors will have to work in shifts to provide adequate medical care.

- House officers are the first line in the medical team, and are usually responsible for the day-to-day care of patients (under supervision), and the organisation of investigations and treatment. Communication with patients and their relatives is a crucial part of the role. The SHO provides support and back-up to this role.

- The type of job and its location depends on matching personal preferences with the opportunities that exist within your chosen Foundation Programme.

- Being a new doctor is one of the toughest years of your life. It can be disruptive of your personal life and emotionally demanding. It can also show teamwork at its best, be great training, good fun, and immensely fulfilling.

11

Developing your career

For as long as there are sick people around there will always be a need for doctors (and undertakers). One of the attractive features of a medical career in the UK has traditionally been the near-guarantee of full employment for the rest of your working life. A decade of reforms in the NHS, the expansion of medical school places and streamlined systems of training for junior doctors has reduced this certainty at least at bottle necks in the career structure. However, despite current challenges for newly qualified doctors the prospect of stable employment still holds true for the overwhelming majority of new doctors. This is not unconditional. You will need to remain competent to practise, keep up to date with medical advances and adhere to the standards of professional practice laid down by the profession's governing body, the General Medical Council (GMC). Another attractive feature of medicine is the surprising variety of jobs which you could consider after your early medical training. For every young medical school applicant who proudly declares at his interview that he intends to pursue a career in neurosurgery, there are perhaps 20 others who know only that they want to be a doctor and as yet have no real idea the precise form that ambition will take. Some will end up delivering babies (obstetricians) while others dissect dead bodies (pathologists), some will care for patients with rare inherited disorders (clinical geneticists) while others work on preventing diseases which affect whole populations (public health physicians). For some doctors, this career uncertainty remains well into their first few years after qualifying. The streamlining of training, bringing it more into line with North American and European programmes, may also mean less

> flexibility than before as new doctors have to commit to career choices earlier on. However, doctors being as they are, no doubt those determined enough to plough their own furrow will soon find ways of doing so while still progressing their career.

The career path

While it is apparent that many new doctors are keen to find innovative ways of developing their career, the "powers that be" (the Department of Health, the Postgraduate Medical Education Training Board, the GMC, and the medical Royal Colleges) have increasingly tried to create more structured training and consistent quality of experience for junior doctors. More systematic training with better supervision, assessment of the skills being developed,

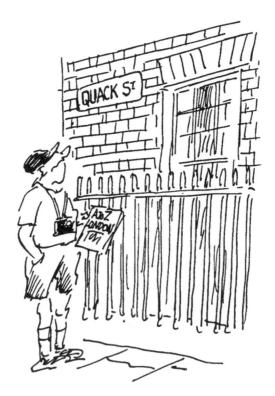

and documentation of the outcomes of each doctor's learning actually allows a degree of flexibility that the old-fashioned "just serve your time and watch me" apprenticeships of former generations lacked. Reforms have been instituted at almost every grade of the medical hierarchy and in all specialities and these will continue to evolve.

A specialist indeed!

Every doctor becomes a specialist, even in something as general sounding as general practice, perhaps better called Family Medicine (as in the USA), which is as much a special art as any other part of medical practice. Becoming a specialist may not seem that difficult, judged from recent cases of bogus doctors who have remained undetected for years. A 64-year-old man with a stolen medical degree was sentenced at Leeds Crown Court after working for 30 years as a general practitioner (GP). Amazingly, neither his patients (some of whom demonstrated outside the court house in his support), nor his colleagues rumbled him. A pharmacist in the chemist's shop next door to the surgery raised the alarm, not perhaps before time. "If one 5 millilitre spoonful of hair shampoo is to be taken orally three times a day", the pharmacists told the court, "You tend to think something is wrong. Time and again there were inhalers to be injected, tablets to be rubbed in, all very unusual". Very unusual!

General practice is not the only home of bogus doctors. Amaedeo Goria of Canelli near Turin practised for 13 years as a neurologist before he was "unwittingly betrayed by his adoring wife after telling her one lie too many about his professional prowess". She passed on to a local newspaper his story that he had brilliantly passed an examination in Rome, which qualified him to become head of the neurology department at the local hospital. This news sparked off an enquiry which revealed to the contrary that he was a failed medical student who had forged his diploma. It could be said that both the public and profession need their gullible heads examined, but they would be wise to take care over who does it. About the same time as Signor Goria was unmasked, another failed medical student in Italy was discovered, not because of clinical incompetence but because of "corruption in appointing senior medical personnel". He had practised for 10 years as a neurosurgeon without detection.

Postgraduate medical education

The Postgraduate Medical Education and Training Board in conjunction with the medical Royal Colleges and related specialist faculties determine the standards of practice and education in the specialities. They inspect and assess both training programmes and placements in conjunction with the Postgraduate Deanery of the local university. A syllabus outlines the broad areas of knowledge, skills and attitudes required. Regular assessments by consultants nominated as clinical supervisors or tutors check the doctor's progress. Examinations for membership or fellowship of a Royal College are taken, now as part of specialist training. Many doctors also take a higher university degree – MD or DM (Doctor of Medicine) awarded for a dissertation which is usually based on clinical research in the course of postgraduate training. Increasingly many other doctors are undertaking Masters level degrees (Master of Science, Master of Public Health, Master of Surgery, or even Masters in Law or Business Administration) at some point in their career either as part of their training or to pursue a related interest later in their career. There are also a host of diplomas which can be taken from various medical Royal Colleges or universities. This is common amongst many GPs who may want to supplement their family practice with a specialist interest in say Child Health, Family Planning, Dermatology or Geriatric Medicine.

Improving working lives

Medicine as a career in the UK is inextricably linked to the National Health Service (NHS) which since its inception in 1948 has been, by far, the main employer of junior doctors and of hospital consultants. A different arrangement is in place for most GPs who are, in effect, self-employed but contracted to provide a service by the NHS. The NHS must, however, continue to be an attractive employment option for qualified doctors, particularly at present where public demand for and commitment to the NHS is leading to a significant expansion in the number of doctors needed across the country. This is occurring at a time when an increasing number of doctors, mainly but not exclusively women, are choosing to work part-time, at least for some of their career. In addition the European Union's employment directives are also forcing the NHS to be a more flexible employer, working for better conditions for staff and encouraging better working conditions (including shorter working hours) than was traditionally endured by most doctors, particularly in their early careers. While it remains true that in many ways being a doctor is more than just a job but a way of life, keeping medicine in its place can be difficult. Dr Julian Eyers when a recent graduate referred to: "… a public misconception that doctors are some sort of breed apart of medical soldiers, ready to be drafted into any situation. Doctors are actually human beings. They have loved ones, emotions, and outside lives".

Not only a parent or carer or elderly relatives, but also the dedicated sportsman, musician, or enthusiast for a full life may wonder whether an otherwise attractive career would unacceptably monopolise their lives. Given the structure of society and the traditionally predominant responsibility of the mother for the family, many of the issues particularly affect women in medicine, but increasing numbers of men have family responsibilities too. And an increasing number of both genders just want to achieve a better work-life balance.

Becoming a thoroughly fulfilled doctor is compatible with domestic commitments provided both partners are prepared to fully share the task of house and home. The trouble is that more than half of married doctors are themselves married to doctors, with all the difficulty that entails, including coordinating training programmes and eventually obtaining mutually compatible career posts. Past studies have shown that half of women and a quarter of men considered marriage to have been a constraint on their career in medicine. Eventually preconceived ambitions have to be balanced against the practicalities of personal commitments and professional training. In this, the medical profession is by no means unique.

To tackle some of these challenges, however, a programme known as *Improving Working Lives* has been established. This aims to increase opportunities for flexible training schemes and flexible career development, improve childcare provision, tackle discrimination and invest a diverse workforce which better reflects the society it serves.

The *Flexible Career Scheme* for doctors (other than GPs who have a different although similar scheme) is designed to allow you to work part-time and to afford some level of choice with how and when you work. Obviously the NHS has to ensure that it is able to staff the service it needs to provide but it should take the rights of its employees into account. There is little doubt that those doctors who wish to work more flexibly are better able to now than previous generations. But, as many parents who wish to work only part-time while they have a young family will testify, it is not always easy to fight your way through the bureaucracy to achieve what is your right.

The Flexible Training Scheme requires those doctors still in training to fulfil at least 50% of their time commitment (usually 5–8 sessions a week, each session being half a day) with a proportional amount of out-of-hour commitment. The overall length of training for all doctors in any speciality is always the same and, understandably, the same competency standards apply so, for instance a psychiatrist who trains part-time while also bringing up a family may spend 7 or 8 years as a part-time specialist registrar before being awarded her CCST and becoming a consultant.

Despite initiatives such as these, there are several medical specialities which remain more popular choices for those who wish to better balance their home and work lives. General practice is often more compatible with other responsibilities, both in terms of flexibility of working practice and in the earlier attainment of a settled home and secure income. Paediatrics, psychiatry, pathology, radiology, and public health are fields which attract high proportions of women applicants.

The NHS is committed to being an equal opportunities employer and states that its entire staff should be treated equitably and fairly with a good quality of working life regardless of age, race, religion, gender or sexual orientation.

Specialist training programmes

On completion of the Foundation Programme, the new doctor then has to make one of the most central decisions of their career development. The application system for this choice is currently under review. The previous scheme was through the online national Medical Training Applications Service (MTAS) for a specialist training programme (a run-through training grade lasting 3–8 years depending on choice of speciality to a senior medical appointment – consultant specialist or general practice principal).

The system ran into troubles with many complaining about the lack of posts, poorly designed recruitment forms and technical failures with the official application website. Junior doctors were angry about the way everyone was made to apply for training schemes at the same time, rather than the old rolling recruitment process which allowed them to apply as and when training posts arose. The over-involvement of politicians was highlighted and the ensuing furore forced the government to take a U-turn. These are described in more detail further on in the chapter. An alternative to entering the specialist training system straight after the Foundation years is to "tread water" while considering your options and apply for a year-long Fixed Term Specialist Training Post.

The second main choice of option is between hospital-based speciality such as gastroenterology or surgery, and a community based specialty such as general practice or public health. This distinction increasingly relates more to the focus of the training years rather than the future location of clinical service delivery as many traditional hospital-based specialists (such as dermatologists, radiologists, genitourinary physicians and even orthopaedic surgeons are spending more of their time seeing patients outside hospitals such as in community clinics or diagnostic and treatment centres.

Once embarked on run-through specialist training programme, the doctor progresses through posts labelled ST1, ST2 (specialist trainee year 1 and 2) etc. The length of training depends on the choice of specialty, with GP training lasting 3–4 years and training for some highly specialised surgeons lasting longer. The details of what competencies are expected to be developed during each phase of training and the exposure to varying clinical areas depends greatly on the programme chosen, but usually starts more general and becomes increasingly specialised as it progresses.

It is usually during this time that the specialist training doctor will add to their knowledge base with the necessary practical skills for their field, such as gastroenterologists learning endoscopy (cameras up and down various orifices), surgeons learning their techniques of increasingly complicated operations, or psychiatrists learning techniques such as psychotherapy.

Many specialist trainees will also undertake some teaching of more junior staff and also medical students where the hospital is attached to a medical school. Some move more definitely into the academic field, becoming a Clinical Lecturer within a university department combining teaching and research with some clinical experience.

Doctors successfully completing a specialty training programme will receive a Certificate of Completion of Training (CCT) and become eligible for entry to the GMC General Practice/Specialist Register. This will then allow then to apply for a senior medical appointment.

Recent difficulties and revolting doctors

Governments have a record for making a mess of major new initiatives which rely on big national IT schemes and the new on-line application system for medical training posts (known as MTAS, Medical Training Application Service) is no exception. It is difficult to find anyone who will defend the system, and so disillusioned have some junior doctors become that they recently took to the streets on protest marches. The government itself has ordered a review and the Secretary of State has been forced to issue a public apology after a series of recent scandals. The system overloading and crashing on the first weekend it was launched (when else would junior doctors find the time to log on?). The site security failed leaving personal details of applicants such as names, phone numbers, and even sexual orientation available to view on-line by the general public, Perhaps most controversially, though there has been an overall feeling from all sections of the medical profession that the anonymous scoring system was incapable of differentiating the quality of candidates, favouring the mediocre and penalising the better applicants. On the first round of applications, of the junior doctors actually able to submit an application, many of the first-rate applicants found themselves without an interview and facing an enforced career break.

There was limited affection for the old system of choosing who got what job – it was often accused of discriminating against women and ethnic minority candidates, it was uncoordinated, time-consuming and lacked fairness and transparency – so we all must hope that the teething troubles of this new scheme are resolved quickly to ensure that a successful medical career can be developed on merit and not as the result of a lottery. From 2008 onwards, it seems recruitment rounds will be CV-based and held on a medical deanery level (e.g. North-Western, East Anglian, London, etc.) instead of a national one. This seems to be more fair, less controversial and certainly allows minimal room for computer error!

Fixed term specialist training appointments

Depending on your point of view these one year posts in a speciality can be thought of as a useful way to continue in an approved training post while delaying a run-through programme while you decided exactly what you want to do, or they can be used to mop up those post-Foundation year doctors who fail to be selected for their chosen job, thereby putting qualified doctors to good use and saving the government the embarrassment of hundreds of unemployed doctors.

They are generally equivalent to ST1 and ST2 posts and will allow you to develop appropriate competencies to that level. From here you can apply to a run-through training programme or side-step to a Career Grade post if you fulfil the necessary requirements.

Career grade posts

In recent years up to a quarter of all NHS hospital doctors have been employed in non-consultant and non-training grade posts providing valuable, but hugely variable, service to the healthcare system. As a group these doctors all too often lacked professional respect partly because of inconsistent skill levels and the fact that they could be employed by individual hospitals on local contracts often paying them considerably less than consultant colleagues despite sometimes minimal difference in what job they actually performed. These posts, previously given fancy titles like Associate Specialists, or Staff Grade Doctors, or Clinical Fellows, are also now subject to more streamlined training requirements and entitled to improved terms and conditions of employment. Such doctors only work in secondary care (not general practice) and have undergone at least 3 years' postgraduate training before appointment. Like any other doctor, they are subject to the same requirements of continuous professional development and regular appraisal.

Becoming a consultant

After obtaining the CCT, doctors compete for a consultant post. Insofar as the term implies simply giving advice to others rather than hands-on examination and treatment as part of a team, the term is outdated and mis-leading. Currently, the relationship between consultant vacancies and the number of specialist trainees nearing the end of the training differs greatly between specialities. In most specialities newly qualified specialists have no difficulty obtaining a consultant post, particularly if they are pre-pared to travel to another part of the country. However, those with family or other commitments anchoring them to particular part of the country can sometimes find the transition from training grade to consultant less than seamless, especially if they are also trying to balance home and work commitments. This will present an every growing challenge to those responsible for medical workforce planning in the future.

Most consultants remain in the same post for many years, developing their practice and moulding the service they provide to the ever-changing demands of modern practice. Some do change posts to move to a different hospital, perhaps to suit family commitments or just to vary the job they do. Some take on additional responsibilities such as becoming involved in the management of the hospital by being a medical director of a hospital

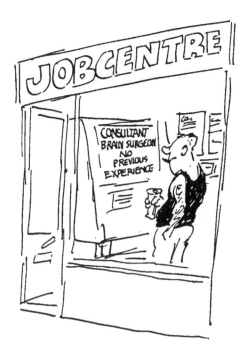

trust, or work with the pharmaceutical industry or with a medical charity. Doctors who have taken their specialist training in academic departments often continue in university hospitals as senior lecturers (with honorary consultant status). In due course, senior lecturers may be promoted to reader or professor.

The NHS currently does not have different levels of seniority of consultant but it does reward exceptional service and scientific distinction with merit awards, salary supplements which can be substantial in relation to the basic salary.

Consultants may undertake private practice alongside their NHS responsibilities. New consultant contracts stipulate exactly what the NHS expects from each consultant through their mutually agreed job plans setting out detailed programmed activities. The myth of the consultant calling his junior doctor to check up on his NHS patients while driving between the golf course and his private consulting rooms is even less true than it has ever been.

Becoming a GP

Most GPs have worked for between 3 and 5 years in hospitals before they move to the health centre or GP surgery. A few spend considerably longer following the hospital specialist career path before deciding to side-step into family practice. Mirroring the changes to other specialities, the training period for general practice has become more structured. GP training schemes are ready-made packages of rotating clinical posts and education. Most currently last three years and include two years in approved hospital-based speciality training posts and one year as a GP Registrar working in a practice under the supervision of an approved senior GP trainer. Some doctors create their own training schemes but it is imperative that all posts have been approved for GP training. The Postgraduate Medical Education and Training Board (www.pmetb.org.uk) can advise further on the regulations relating to approved training posts. Some schemes are extending the length of time spent as a GP Registrar either by extending the overall training to 3½ or 4 years, while others divide the 3 years equally between training posts in hospitals and general practice.

The commonest hospital posts to be included in GP training include general medicine, care of the elderly, paediatrics, obstetrics and gynaecology, psychiatry, accident and emergency, and specialities such as dermatology, rheumatology, ophthalmology, and ear, nose, and throat surgery.

The year as a GP Registrar is usually spent in one approved training practice, though schemes vary the timing of this element of the training with some providing a shorter "taster" attachment at the beginning of the 3-year training to help the would-be GP understand what knowledge and skills they need to develop over the remainder of their training. Each registrar is allocated a GP Trainer, who is themselves an experienced and specially trained GP, in whose practice the attachment is provided and who supervises the clinical work and educational development of the registrar. In addition, it is a well-established element of GP training that a half-day a week throughout the 3 years of the scheme is set aside for an educational session. The nature of these is usually very much down to the doctors themselves to decide with the guidance of an experienced GP Course Organiser.

All GP Registrars must pass the examination for membership of the Royal College of General Practitioners before being awarded their CCT. Once this training is complete and the new GP is accepted onto the general practice register they are free to choose from the many varied models of employment available to GPs ranging from joining an established practice as a full-time partner to being a portfolio GP with the working week divided between various roles including clinical practice, teaching, research, management, or developing a specialist interest such as dermatology or cardiology.

REMEMBER

- Medicine offers relatively secure, well-paid employment in a large variety of possible careers.

- Students should start to consider their career options by their fourth or fifth year at medical school. Many have no firm intentions at this stage beyond knowing a few areas which they have discounted.

- "Flexible" part-time training is possible in most specialities for those for whom full-time training is not practicable.

- All senior medical appointments in the NHS, whether consultants or principals in general practice, need to obtain a Certificate of Completion of Training.

- An increasing number of junior doctors spend time out of the NHS, travelling, working abroad, working in a different field or just taking out a gap year. For most this gives them time to settle on their intended career options and keep a healthy perspective on their life, and it is no longer regarded unfavourably by many employers but needs to be timed carefully.

The growing influence of politicians upon medicine has helped and hindered members of the profession. Like it or loathe it, government and medicine are entwined. The reversal of the 2007 MTAS application scheme is evidence that organisations of young doctors like the BMA Junior Doctors Committee, are influential, if they kick up enough of a fuss!

12

Career opportunities

Medicine offers an amazing range of different career options. Most doctors end up in one of the three main areas of general practice, a hospital-based speciality, or public health. Smaller numbers of doctors end up in a huge range of possible careers as varied as military doctors to journalists, coroners to playwrights, pharmaceutical company researchers to missionary hospital doctors, expedition medics to university lecturers. Medical students are well advised to take a careful look at the very broad canvas of opportunity before they qualify. Most people finally choose their speciality within 2 or 3 years of graduation. However an increasing number of doctors attempt to choose careers which are more varied, include other interests, and are flexible enough to allow them to fit their career around their life, not the other way round. This chapter gives a taste of what each speciality is like and illustrates the wide variety of career opportunities open to a newly qualified doctor.

How and when to decide which speciality

Some fortunate people decide on their careers as students (fortunate, that is, if they have made a realistic decision), more decide in the first few years after medical school. Having cleared the hurdles of final examinations and foundation programme, and having found their medical feet in these mostly general posts, most students begin to focus on the speciality which appeals to them. Careers fairs are held annually in many parts of the country to display the attractions and to offer advice from doctors in all major specialities on a personal and informal level. The foundation programme is expected to offer personalised, formal career advice although in reality this is not yet as widespread as it needs to be. The Royal Colleges also appoint local advisers who can be useful sources of advice on the practicalities of the training and opportunities of each speciality. The *British Medical Journal* (bmj.com/careers) also has an extensive careers section in its weekly edition which provides a wide range of descriptions of specialities with personal experiences of doctors in certain fields as well as broader careers advice on topics such as preparing your curriculum vitae (CV) and interview techniques.

At the end of the day, not every doctor ends up in their speciality of first choice because, in the words of George Bernard Shaw: "Up to a point doctors, like carpenters and masons, must earn their living by doing work that the public wants from them". Or, put another way by a former chief medical officer at the Department of Health: "The aim of undergraduate medical education is to produce doctors who are able to meet the present and future needs of the health services".

Remember though, that perfect fits are for machines: more roughly crafted men and women and evolving specialities are seldom made precisely for each other. But if the interest and the will are there, the individual and the speciality can develop together like partners in a successful marriage. Doctor and speciality is not the only fit which matters. Spare a thought for the doctor–patient relationship on the way, bearing in mind Dr Brotschi's snapshots of "the kind of doctors we shouldn't be" in a letter to the *New England Journal of Medicine*:

> First, the ambitious climber take,
> Who will the department chairman make;
> Who toils to win Professors' praise
> And quotes the Journal, phrase by phrase,
> But never reads the patients' gaze.
>
> Next: the expert proud we find,
> The latest saviour to mankind.
> Cured patients speak to his renown,
> But he leaves sick ones with a frown,
> Because they let his image down.

Third, the jovial friend of all,
Who never heard perfection's call.
His ken of medicine paper thin,
But patients' trust he'll always win:
They love him while he does them in.

And fourth, the well adjusted fellow,
Who seeks that all in life be mellow;
Who loves good music, wine and skis,
Resents his work but likes the fees,
And does not hear his patients' pleas.

To start the series, here are four,
But surely there are many more,
Just let us seek and see what's true
In what we are and what we do,
Lest we forget, we're human too.

General practice

General practice, also known as family medicine, is a demanding but fulfilling career. Along with other professional colleagues (such as nurses, therapists, family dentists, community pharmacists, and optometrists) they form the major "frontline" of the NHS, known as primary care. Together these primary care professionals undertake 90% of all patient consultations within the NHS.

As a new general practitioner (GP) you can choose how many sessions you wish to work each week which allows you greater flexibility to combine being a GP with outside interests such as raising a family or developing skills in research or another clinical area, becoming a GP with a special interest. General practice offers the prospect of a settled home and higher income at an earlier stage than a career in the hospital service. GPs who live (as most do) in the district in which they practise, naturally become very much part of their local community and have the satisfaction of giving long-term continuity of care, often looking after several generations of families from "the cradle to the grave". For many GPs this hugely privileged role offers the unique attraction of the speciality. In some instances this continuity of care aspect is less pronounced if you chose to practise in an inner city where a higher proportion of the population is continuously changing and where as many as a third of your patients may change each year. This may bring its own interests and challenges, however, and many GPs who have had experience of both rural and urban general practice will testify that there are more similarities than differences.

Some GPs also take on clinical leadership roles within their local Primary Care Trust (PCT) or equivalent, or have grouped together with colleagues to hold the main responsibility for commissioning the services of hospital and other health care providers (such as community mental health services) on behalf of the patients registered with local GPs.

Increasingly in addition to their "general" clinical caseload, many GPs are choosing to take on a specialist role with services provided by their local PCT, often in conjunction with the local hospital team. In the future, many patients will be seen in community clinics by a GP specialist rather than be seen by a hospital specialist. These services are already commonly provided for clinical areas with high demand for second opinions such as dermatology, ear, nose, and throat surgery, family planning and sexual health, gastroenterology, asthma, allergies, low back pain, and drug and alcohol services.

There is increasing flexibility of employment arrangements as well. The majority of GPs still work in partnership in a practice with other GPs, though large numbers of sole practitioner practices exist especially in inner-city areas. These doctors are contracted to provide general medical services for a list of patients (approximately 1500 patients for each GP) and they earn a profit on this business which they take as their salary. However, many new GPs choose to work for these practices (as salaried employees) rather than as a partner in the business, at least for a few years. This type of job carries the same clinical commitment (and means you are no less qualified as a GP) but leaves greater flexibility if, for instance, family or other work circumstances require it. Gradually, however, most GPs settle in a practice for some time and build up the continuing care relationship with their patients.

Opportunities exist for part-time work and many GPs combine their clinical commitments with family responsibilities or other roles such as teaching medical students, research or management. GPs no longer have the contractual commitment to provide for 24-hour care for their patients; this is now the responsibility of the PCT (or equivalent) instead. Patients must still be able to get to see a doctor whenever they need to, so some doctors will choose to work anti-social hours at nights and weekends to cover these services. Some will do so because of a sense of duty and some because of the high rates of pay on offer (and some for a bit of both reasons).

Like all medical careers, general practice fluctuates in popularity with medical graduates, but with increasing flexibility, a range of opportunities, and a new contract bringing improved pay and conditions for many GPs, it is currently undergoing a renaissance of popularity and esteem. From 2008 all doctors wishing to work as a GP in the UK must appear on the GMC's GP Register. To achieve this you must complete an approved training scheme which includes passing the examination of Membership of the Royal College of General Practitioners.

Accident and emergency

People with acute injuries or sudden acute illness often dial 999 for the ambulance service, are picked up from the street, or are urgently sent to hospital by their doctor. Others taken less acutely or seriously ill, who for one reason or another do not call their GP, take themselves straight to hospital. Many accident and emergency departments include both a minor injuries unit run entirely by nurse practitioners and the consultant led medical team who provide for the patients requiring acute resuscitation, full medical assessment, or more complicated medical treatment. A&E Departments also play a central role in the emergency response to major incidents such as train crashes or terrorist attacks. Such incidents may happen only rarely but all departments have to have well-rehearsed plans ready to be enacted at a few minutes' notice. The consultants are in overall charge of the whole team, but the initial sorting of cases is the responsibility of an experienced nurse who also ensures appropriate destination and priority for each individual.

Dealing with anything and everything serious, not so serious, or difficult to discern requires special skill, training, and experience, useful whatever medical speciality a doctor eventually ends up in. For that reason, many senior house officer training programmes in medicine, surgery, and several other specialities now include a period of several months in the accident and emergency department to develop this core dimension of practical professional skill. Telling the difference between the apparently trivial and a medical or surgical time bomb is an art fully learnt only through active service in front-line trenches; getting it right, or at least not sending the patient home without fail-safe follow-up, can save tens of lives and hundreds of thousands of pounds in medical litigation fees and damages.

Accident and emergency consultants have in the past usually had a background in surgery, medicine, anaesthetics, or general practice and have obtained qualifications related to those specialties. Specific training programmes now exist leading to becoming a Fellow of the College of Emergency Medicine (FCEM). Accident and emergency is one of the few clinical specialities which readily lends itself to shift working. Most patients are treated and referred back to their GPs so there is little call for continuity of care. Learning from experience is assured by regular meetings of the whole team to review successes and failures.

Anaesthetics

Anaesthetics is another speciality in which continuity of care is limited: preoperative assessment, the operation itself, the early recovery period, and intermittent periods of responsibility for supervising the intensive care unit. It is a very hands-on speciality and if you are up all night provision is normally made for you to be off for at least part of the next day. The work of an anaesthetist falls fairly tidily into regular and carefully defined commitments.

Providing pain relief or anaesthesia during surgical operations, childbirth, and diagnostic procedures is the major task of an anaesthetist. Some anaesthetists also specialise further and run clinics for people with chronic pain, and a new Faculty of Pain Medicine has been incorporated by the Royal College of Anaesthetists to recognise this growing field of expertise. Many consultants also take turns in charge of the intensive care unit, though an increasing number confine themselves to such work. In time, it is expected that a further specialist faculty will take the lead in the field of intensive care medicine, following the example of Australia and New Zealand who have had a well-established faculty for some years. Anaesthetics is a large and expanding speciality.

The primary examination for Fellowship of the Royal College of Anaesthetists (FRCAnaes) can be taken 18 months after graduation, usually taken during a senior house officer post in anaesthetics, and is a test of knowledge of the scientific basis of anaesthetics and anaesthesia. The final part of the FRCAnaes is taken during the later stages of specialist training.

Medicine

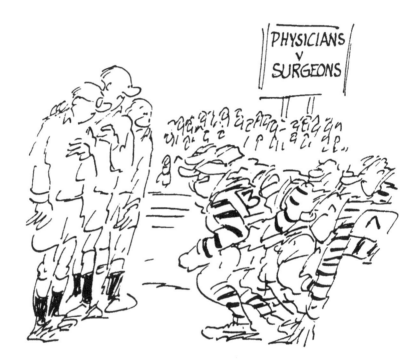

Specialists in medicine in the UK are known as "physicians". On the whole, medicine and surgery attract different personalities: physicians tend to be more reflective; surgeons more executive. The difference is reflected in the respective Royal Colleges as Dr John Rowan Wilson observed some years ago but nothing much has changed:

The Royal Colleges are, of course, much the smarter end of the profession; they represent the big time. However, the two main colleges, the Physicians and the Surgeons, are very different in character. The Royal College of Physicians, like the Catholic Church, is ancient and obscurely hierarchical. It occupies a tiny Vatican in Regents Park, whose benign soft-footed cardinals pad around discussing preferment of one kind or another. To be a Member of the College (achieved by examination) counts for nothing at all.

One must be elected a Fellow. ... In turning to the College of Surgeons one moves from the episcopal to the military. Surgeons are brash, extrovert characters who pride themselves on energy rather than subtlety. Fellowship is decided by examination, and theoretically all Fellows are equal, just as theoretically all officers are gentlemen.

Some physicians are specialists in a subject such as dermatology (skin diseases) or rheumatology (joint and muscle disorders) but most have dual certification in general medicine and a subspeciality. "Internal" is sometimes added to the title of general medicine because that is the North American term for the speciality.

The "general" label, means that the physician can successfully bat any acute medical emergency balls, at least hitting them towards an appropriate fielder. In practice, this requires the ability to cope with any and every acute medical emergency, at least in the initial stage, and the ability to deal with unstructured diagnostic problems not falling obviously into any particular subspeciality at an early stage. Most British hospitals are not large enough either to have a specialist in each subspeciality of medicine or to maintain an acute medical emergency rota for patients who need to be admitted to hospital at any hour of the day or night without the participation of most of the specialist physicians. The position is similar in surgery.

Time and again, hospital specialist practice requires well-informed clinical common sense rather than intensely specialised knowledge. Prof. J. R. A. Mitchell told the story of a patient who reappeared in his outpatient clinic, having being referred from specialist to specialist, saying, "there is no point in sending me to another specialist, doctor, it is not my special parts which have gone wrong but what holds them together". That sentiment notwithstanding the growing sub-specialisation of medicine continues with even the smallest hospitals have more consultants in specialist fields such as cardiology, endocrinology and diabetes, gastroenterology, sexual health, neurology, renal and respiratory medicine.

Membership of the Royal Colleges of Physicians of the United Kingdom (MRCP (UK)) is the professional diploma needed before you complete specialist training. The Royal Colleges of Physicians in London and Edinburgh, and the Royal College of Physicians and Surgeons in Glasgow hold a common membership examination. Election to fellowship normally follows about 10 years after passing the examination for membership.

The MRCP diploma part 1 (written exam) is a necessary entry qualification to the later stages specialist training and part 2 (written and clinical exam) is usually completed during the third or fourth specialist training years. Although the examination is difficult and the pass rate is low, more doctors are successful in the examination than can become specialists in medicine. Some deliberately acquire the diploma as an additional qualification before entering another hospital speciality or general practice. The MRCP examination is, above all, a test of clinical skills: it covers similar ground to the final MB examination in medicine but at a more demanding and discriminating level. It is necessary to know about rarities but it is even more important to have sound clinical skill and common sense, based on expertise in managing everyday medical emergencies.

Paediatrics and child health

The care of children, especially of the newborn, has become immensely specialised. Forty years ago, paediatrics was part of general medicine, but not now. The skills required are very different from those required in adult medicine and so too is the spectrum of disease. The special nature of paediatrics, its role, and range across the divide between hospital and community, and the interplay of medical, psychiatric, and social factors in child care was finally and formally recognised by the founding of the Royal College of Paediatrics and Child Health in 1996, which has developed its own membership examination.

Paediatric subspecialities are still less well developed than those in adult medicine and practically all paediatricians working at any but the very largest and most specialised hospitals need to participate also in a general emergency service, either in neonatal intensive care, acute paediatrics, or child protection. Increasing some paediatricians choose to work outside of hospitals in the community and work closely with schools and GPs in providing specialist advice to children and families in conjunction with specialist nurses and therapists and their hospital-based colleagues. Paediatrics is a speciality in which consultants have a particularly large hands-on involvement in the acute emergency work. Specialist training is likewise very practically intensive. Children become seriously ill very quickly and, with immediate intervention, can improve just as fast.

Obstetrics and gynaecology

Obstetrics and gynaecology is one speciality with two different aspects. Obstetrics offers a balance between medicine and surgery with the attraction of usually young and healthy patients, and a happy outcome to the encounter. Gynaecology (diseases specifically of women) also demands both surgical and medical skills. There are still posts which combine these two areas in equal measure, particularly in district general hospitals but increasingly consultants tend to develop, in addition, a subspecialist interest; for example, in the investigation and treatment of sub-fertility, the management of the menopause or contraception, urogynaecology (combining conditions of the bladder and reproductive organs) or community sexual health.

Specialists in this field become Members of the Royal College of Obstetricians and Gynaecologists (MRCOG). Part I of the examination, a multiple-choice paper on the basic sciences, is related to the speciality and may be taken at any time after full registration. Part II is taken after at least 3 years in approved posts and includes written, clinical, and oral examinations, together with preparation of case records and commentaries. Instruction in family planning is included in the training. Some obstetricians train first in general surgery and obtain the Membership of a Royal College of Surgeons (MRCS) to acquire a much wider surgical ability than their limited surgical speciality necessarily demands; a few start in medicine (particularly endocrinology) and first pass the MRCP; an occasional brilliant workhorse obtains both these diplomas and the MRCOG.

Pathology

If television dramas painted a complete picture of medical specialties then the public would be forgiven for believing at least half the doctors in the country must work in forensic pathology (and therefore spend their life solving crimes by cutting up dead bodies washed up on picturesque riversides and having affairs with the chief suspects). In reality, the specialities within pathology provide a wide range of laboratory diagnostic services which are an essential part of everyday clinical practice and the forensic pathologist is a rare (but necessary) breed of pathologist with a highly specialised area of morbid expertise. The clinical biochemist is an expert in the biochemical mechanisms and diagnosis of disease; the histopathologist and cytologist is an expert in diagnosing disease from changes in tissue or cell structure; and the medical microbiologist (a title which includes bacteriologist, virologist, and mycologist) is an expert in the culture and identification of bacteria, viruses, fungi, and other communicable causes of disease. Some medical microbiologists combine this diagnostic function with the detection, epidemiological monitoring, and control of outbreaks of infection, based in one of the laboratories of the Health Protection Agency.

The haematologist is concerned with disorders of the blood (such as leukaemia) and with blood transfusion; some haematologists specialise entirely in blood transfusion and work for the National Blood Transfusion Service. Clinical immunology is a small but expanding speciality which spans laboratory science and clinical medicine. It is concerned particularly with the role of immune reactions in disease.

Although based in the laboratory, pathologists are often consulted about patients at their colleagues' request. The medical microbiologist, for example, should be in a position to give expert advice on antibiotic treatment of serious infections and on the control of the spread of infections in hospital. Haematologists normally have patients under their care in wards and outpatients. Besides having scientific and clinical skills, the consultant pathologist needs to be capable of becoming a good director of a laboratory.

For a career in all these pathology specialities, with the exception of clinical immunology for which the MRCP may be more appropriate and haematology for which it is customary to have both memberships, it is necessary to become a Member of the Royal College of Pathologists (MRCPath). The part I examination is taken after 3 years in one of the many specialities of pathology. It is no longer a test of all branches of pathology. Part II is taken at a minimum of 2 years after part I and is limited to the chosen speciality.

Psychiatry

Psychiatry is an expanding speciality which is changing rapidly, not least because new treatments are substantially reducing the need for inpatient treatment, especially the need for long stay mental hospitals. Political policy has also moved many long-term psychiatric patients out of hospital into a community which unfortunately cannot always cope with them or they with the community. Psychiatry includes the subspeciality of mental handicap, a Cinderella subject with the task of deploying a range of medical and engineering skills, together with human insight to help handicapped patients realise their own potential. The emphasis in their care is shifting towards rehabilitation in small units before they attempt to return to their own homes.

The examination for Membership of the Royal College of Psychiatrists (MRCPsych) may be taken after a minimum of 3 years of specialist training. This means working as a specialist training doctor in a psychiatric hospital looking after both emergency and long stay patients, besides seeing patients in the psychiatric outpatient clinic and in community-based services such as rapid response teams which can be called to assess patients with acute severe mental health problems. It is possible to specialise in either adult or child psychiatry but all psychiatrists are expected to have some experience of both.

A good knowledge of medicine is valuable in psychiatry, and some psychiatrists acquire the MRCP in the early years of their training.

Diagnostic radiology

Like pathologists, radiologists need to be good organisers because sooner or later they are likely to have to manage all or part of a department. They need to be skilled with their hands in performing invasive investigations, such as cannulation of internal vessels and biopsy of deep-seated lumps under screening, and in interventional techniques, such as angioplasty (dilatation of narrow blood vessels). They also need to be sharp with their eyes and quick with their brains in interpreting X-ray films and scans. Responsibility for radioisotope investigations normally also falls within the responsibility of the radiologist. Many radiologists obtain the MRCP or occasionally the FRCS while gaining clinical experience before taking up radiology. Diagnostic radiology serves all clinical departments and often provides an open access service for GPs as well. Advances in radiology, particularly computerised scanning, have transformed clinical practice in many specialities. Radiologists therefore have a natural link with most of their colleagues. They also have contact with patients but without overall clinical responsibility for their treatment. Out-of-hour duties are generally not heavy with the exception of subspecialities such as neuroradiology.

Fellowship of the Royal College of Radiologists (FRCR) is a necessary qualification. Part I is taken after at least 1 year in a recognised specialist training post and part II after at least 3 years of training.

Oncology

Cancer is treated by radiotherapy, drugs, and surgery. Treatment of cancer by irradiation (radiotherapy) or by drugs (chemotherapy). Oncologists often develop expertise in one particular modality but increasingly these treatments undertake overlapping and so does the training of oncologists and their subsequent clinical workload. Successful treatment of cancer requires teamwork and oncologists not only work closely with multi-disciplinary teams to support the patient through their treatment but also with other specialities, especially with surgeons, physicians, and gynaecologists.

Surgery

Surgery was once considered a craft rather than as a now well-established intellectual and practical art. Surgical specialities are, in a manner of speaking, more cut and dried than medical specialities, as Henri de Mondeville observed in the 13th century:

Surgery is superior to Medicine, because among other things it is more lucrative. To receive gifts or money, a surgeon dare not fear stench, must be able to cut like an executioner, politely lie and be clever. ... The sick above all want to be cured; the surgeon to be paid.

A surgeon is often portrayed, especially in television dramas, as always dressed in theatre gowns, nurse mopping his brow (though a few women surgeons have been portrayed on television, usually as far more fierce than any man would dare be), performing some death-defying feat. Although there is, of course, an element of this, surgeons also hold outpatient clinics, clinical meetings (such as with colleagues in pathology and radiology), and see patients on ward rounds for as much (if not more) of their time than they spend in the operating theatre. The procedures used by surgeons have become increasingly precise and the use of minimally invasive (keyhole) techniques continues to be developed.

Surgical training tends to start with gaining experience in more general areas of the speciality. The MRCS examination is taken at the end of the first stage of surgical training. The trainee then moves into their later specialist training which provides training in both general surgery and a subspeciality, although there are growing trends to concentrate on the specialist element such as becoming an ear, nose, and throat (ENT) or eye (ophthalmic) or breast surgeon. Towards the end of this period of surgical specialist training there is a further examination, the FRCS, which is an examination run by the four surgical colleges of Great Britain and Ireland. The examination particularly tests clinical skills and, together with the necessary years of experience, qualifies the trainee for the CCT. Surgeons often obtain dual certification in general surgery and a subspeciality because most consultant surgeons are expected to cover acute surgical emergencies and undertake some relatively unspecialised surgery besides having a special field of expertise.

Sports and exercise medicine

In 2006 the UK medical Royal Colleges agreed to set up a new Faculty of Sports and Exercise Medicine (SEM). This followed a decision by the Department of Health to recognise SEM as a full medical speciality following the successful introduction of similar changes in Australia and New Zealand. The field is primarily concerned with eth effects of sport and exercise on health including health promotion and also including prevention and treatment of sports-related injuries. The new speciality is very much in its infancy and there remains much uncertainty about the future scale of development of the specialty in the NHS, although the impending London Olympics in 2012 is being seen as an obvious catalyst for the development of the specialism.

Public health medicine

Public health is the medical speciality which is concerned with the improvement of the health of populations – by health promotion and disease prevention, and supporting the commissioning of high quality, cost effective health care from providers of health care, mainly hospitals and GPs. Public health doctors work closely with doctors in many specialities and with other health professionals, with managers, and with government and voluntary organisations. Public health recognises that health requires more than individual patient care. If all members of society are to achieve a better and more equitable health status and health experience, collective action is essential.

It is worth remembering that public health doctors have had every bit as great, if not greater, impact on improving health than physicians and surgeons. A tablet to William Henry Duncan, Medical Officer of Health of Liverpool, who died in 1863, records that "… under the blessing of God he succeeded in reducing the rate of mortality in Liverpool by nearly one third". Epidemiology, the discipline concerned with describing and explaining the occurrence of disease in populations (originally epidemics of infectious disease) and of the outcome of measures to improve health and prevent disease, is the science fundamental to public health medicine and indeed to a substantial proportion of modern medical research. Public health doctors also require a range of other skills, most crucially those associated with management, interpersonal, and political skills in representing the need for more resources for health care and for better use of them.

Public health physicians work in a number of settings within the NHS, the university, central government, and national agencies, such as the Health Protection Agency.

The professional qualification if the examination for Membership of the Faculty of Public Health (MFPH of the Royal College of Physicians of London), which covers epidemiology, statistics, social and behavioural sciences, the principles of prevention of disease and promotion of health, assessment of health needs and audit of services provided, environmental health, and the management and organisation of health services. It is a rapidly expanding speciality. During the years of specialist training, the trainee in public health medicine will often undertake a Master degree and be expected to write a report on practical projects as part of the requirement for part II of the MFPH examination.

Other specialities

Clinical academic medicine

A degree of creative tension often exists between the NHS consultants and clinical academic (university) staff, well expressed by the Royal Commission on Medical Education in 1968:

> There are still full-time academic teachers who see the part-timer as a prosperous busy practitioner who owes his success to clinical acumen rather than painstaking investigation, whose teaching is based on personal dogma rather than scientific fact and whose interests require the whims of private patients to take priority over the needs of his students. There are still part-time teachers who see the full-timer as a desiccated preacher more interested in the advancement of medicine than in the welfare of his patients and unable to offer his students any guidance to the realities of life outside the ivory tower.

There is a smattering of truth in each perspective to the extent that the clinical academic physician or surgeon was described by Dean Holly Smith as "an uneasy hybrid who constantly feels attenuated at both ends".

An academic career in university posts is possible in practically all hospital specialities, general practice, and public health, though the number of posts is small. Clinical senior lecturers, readers, and professors all normally have NHS consultant responsibilities, but they generally have less clinical service work and relatively more time than NHS consultants for teaching and research.

Basic medical sciences

It is widely but not universally believed that medical students benefit from being taught anatomy, physiology, biochemistry, and pharmacology by medical graduates because they best understand the clinical context of these sciences and their relevance to clinical medicine. Few medical graduates, however, now work in these university departments, not least because salaries are lower than those of clinical academics and of other doctors working in the NHS.

Full-time research

A small number of full-time research posts are available to medical graduates, mainly in institutions of the Medical Research Council or in the pharmaceutical industry.

Occupational medicine

Doctors have long been involved in the understanding and preventing of health risks in the workplace but only recently has occupational medicine developed as a clinical speciality rather than as a branch of public health. It includes the former discipline of industrial medicine. The speciality is concerned with identifying and investigating the medical problems associated with different working environments and with advising both management and employees on the prevention of occupational medical hazards.

The examination for Membership of the Faculty of Occupational Medicine (MFOM) of the Royal College of Physicians of London is taken after appropriate training and experience in occupational medicine; a formal specialist training programme leads up to it. Occupational medicine is another speciality suitable for part-time service.

Armed services

The three major branches of the armed services offer careers for both hospital specialists and GPs on long- or short-term contracts. Many doctors begin a service career with a short service commission while they are medical

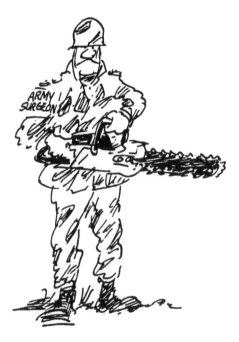

students. In return for a good salary during clinical training and the first foundation year these doctors are required to serve for a further 5 years in the armed services. The armed forces need doctors of all kinds from trauma surgeons to psychiatrists and GPs.

Some doctors who specialise in other fields serve in the reserve forces, such as the Territorial Army, attending regular training and on occasion (such as recent conflicts in Sierra Leone, Iraq and Afghanistan) being called up either on the front-line or to replace regular medical teams sent from military hospitals in the UK.

Pharmaceutical industry

The pharmaceutical industry employs an increasing number of doctors in clinical research and in an advisory capacity. Most doctors entering the industry have a good background in clinical pharmacology or specialist medicine. A new Faculty of Pharmaceutical Medicine exists with membership examinations as recognition of the emerging status and growth in recruitment to this specialism.

Medical journalism

The *British Medical Journal*, the *Lancet*, and a number of other publications have full-time medically qualified editors, together with some who are not medically qualified. Many specialist medical journals have part-time medical editors, as do several newspapers and industry-sponsored medical publications. Freelance opportunities in journalism, radio, and television abound for fluent doctors with lively minds though some are perhaps less high-minded than others: for every Robert Winston prime-time BBC series there's some poor wannabe TV doc talking about teenage sex on a late-night phone-in cable TV channel. And then there's Harry Hill. You might even become a novelist or playwright along with Somerset Maugham, Anton Chekhov, Jed Mercurio, Tim Willocks by dipping your creative pen into your medical life experience.

Voluntary work

Some doctors at all stages of their careers (including a growing number of fit and healthy retired doctors) chose to volunteer their time and experience to charities specialising in providing medical care in the developing world.

Opportunities exist through organisations such as VSO (Voluntary Service Overseas) and MSF (Medecins sans Frontieres) to work in a variety of roles from providing primary care services in war-torn Afghanistan to teaching medical students in Malawi.

REMEMBER

- The broad choice is between hospital-based specialities, general practice, or public health. Most doctors choose their speciality towards the end of their foundation years but around a third will change their mind over the next 3 years, sometimes more than once. The commonest reason for changing choice is personal and family commitments.

- Specialities vary substantially in the amount of emergency work, and therefore in the disruption of personal life.

- Some specialities are more popular than others, and this is ever-changing. It pays to explore all the options.

- Some doctors are able to combine more than one speciality, such as general practice with a special interest in a medical or surgical specialism or public health or medical journalism.

- General practice allows greater continuity of care of families and individuals in a community over a long period. It also offers more flexible working hours, the chance to be "more your own boss", a settled home and a higher income and at an earlier stage.

- The major hospital specialities are accident and emergency, anaesthesia, medical specialities (e.g. cardiology, care of the elderly, gastroenterology, dermatology), obstetrics and gynaecology, paediatrics, psychiatry, pathology, diagnostic radiology, radiotherapy and cancer, ophthalmology, and surgical specialities (e.g. colorectal surgery, orthopaedic surgery, ear/nose/throat surgery).

- Increasing opportunities exist for non-consultant senior grades in some hospital specialities.

- Public health medicine is concerned with the improvement of the health of populations rather than individuals, and with the organisation of health service provision.

- Clinical academic medicine combines specialist training with enhanced opportunities for teaching and research.

- A few doctors follow careers in a variety of other fields, for example, the armed forces, occupational medicine, the pharmaceutical industry, or the media.

13

Privileges and responsibilities: avoiding the pitfalls

> The public is entitled to high professional standards from doctors and it is a privilege to be a doctor. But privileges carry obligations. From the first day that you have contact with patients as a medical student, you carry a personal responsibility and you will be individually accountable. You need to consider carefully whether you are prepared to pay that price, now and for the rest of your professional life.

Paragraph 1 of *Good Medical Practice* published in November 2006 states

Patients need good doctors. Good doctors make the care of their patients their first concern; they are competent, keep their knowledge and skills up to date, establish and maintain good relationships with patients and colleagues, are honest and trustworthy and act with integrity.

It is, of course, purely coincidental that legal issues and the pitfalls of practice are raised in Chapter 13 but the likelihood is that sooner or later, rightly or wrongly, each one of us will be faced with a complaint. This may emanate from a patient, a relative of a patient, an employer, a colleague or from another health professional. Patients have high expectations and you will be much better employed caring for them than dealing with lawyers.

Before making a life choice as to whether medicine is right for you and you are right for medicine, you need to consider whether you have the necessary temperament and resilience to deal with death and disappointment as well as the huge rewards of medicine and also with complaints. It is worth spending time now thinking about some of the less savoury aspects of medical practice and also considering whether there is anything you can do to avoid complaints or to mitigate the consequences to patients and their families and also to yourself.

Unquestionably, there is much that you can do to avoid complaints. Common sense and the principles of good practice should pervade your practice from the very first day that you set foot on a ward or in a general practitioner's (GP's) surgery – that is to say from early in your medical education. Wisdom comes with experience but commonsense should be present from the beginning.

Right from the start you need to make time to ponder upon some of the big issues you may encounter and you should try to sensitise yourself so that you recognise when a tricky situation is looming or has arisen. You need to develop antennae that will tell you when the alarm bells should be starting to ring and, of course, you need to learn not only from your own mistakes but also from the mistakes of others.

It is to be hoped that this book will be useful throughout your training and it may even provoke lively discussion with your seniors! Hopefully, this chapter will not deter you from embarking on a career in medicine but it is important to be realistic and to acquire as much information as you can before making your choice. We hope that it will be bedside reading throughout your professional life, as it aims to provide a useful reminder of some fundamental points it is so easy to lose sight of at stressful times.

In all the professions we live in an era of increased scrutiny and our work is (rightly) constantly under the microscope. Every member of a profession is individually and collectively accountable. Following a number of high profile cases, the public and media have come to question the way doctors have been regarded in the past and their status within society. Doctors now have to earn and maintain public confidence. The public is much readier to hold doctors to account and the standards applied must be acceptable to society as a whole. As Richard Smith (quoting W.B.Yeats) observed in the *British Medical Journal* (*BMJ*) after the Bristol Paediatric Cardiac Surgery case, "All changed, changed utterly". Apart from anything else, it is now well recognised that all doctors including those working in management have a professional responsibility to take action if they believe that the actions of a colleague may be putting patients at risk.

In the fifth report of the Shipman Inquiry published in December 2004, Dame Janet Smith suggested that, although there were signs that the culture

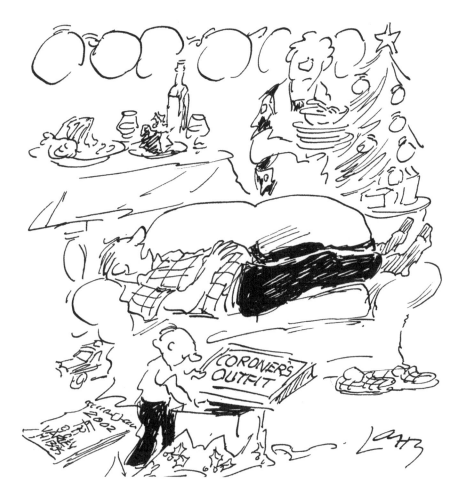

of mutual self-protection had changed, the process was by no means complete. It is vital, she said, "that young doctors are imbued with the new culture from the start. But it is also vital that the leaders of the profession consistently put the message across to the present generation of doctors. There can be no room today for the protection of colleagues where the safety and welfare of patients are at issue."

In December 2004, the Department of Health confirmed its intention to review all the recommendations in the Shipman Report and on 14 July 2006, the Chief Medical Officer (the CMO), Sir Liam Donaldson, published his report entitled "Good doctors, safer patients". In the report he suggests that it is vital to find a universally accepted definition of what constitutes a "good doctor". The GMC have made a stab at this in Good Medical Practice but it may be fruitful for you to consider whether there are further points that could be made. Dressed up in various ways this point must surely feature in many medical school interviews.

The CMO made 44 recommendations in his report and on 21 February 2007, after a lengthy consultation process, the Government published its White Paper entitled "Trust, Assurance and Safety – The Regulation of Health Professionals in the 21st Century". Many of the proposals in that White Paper require either primary or secondary legislation but however matters are carried forward, the message remains constant: patients come first and the quality and safety of patient care must be central to the goals, culture and day-to-day activities of every organisation and every clinical team delivering care to both NHS and private patients. Importantly, it is recognised that the very great majority of doctors provide an excellent and dedicated service to patients. Whilst it is suggested that any changes must bring a more rehabilitative and supportive emphasis to professional regulation, it is difficult to see how that can be reconciled with the climate in which we live and also how such rehabilitation and support will be funded or provided.

Although I hope that it cannot yet be said that we have a "complaints culture" in the UK, the fact is that an increasing number of complaints are made locally and some doctors will receive a letter from the GMC advising them that information has been received which raises a question as to whether their fitness to practise is impaired and therefore about their registration. They should not despair; the end of a short and glorious career is not necessarily nigh.

Very many problems giving rise to complaints are avoidable and almost all complaints can be mitigated. What this chapter aims to do is to highlight a few problem areas, to encourage you to test how resilient you really are, to discourage you from burying your head in the sand and to promote a greater awareness of simple things you can do to avoid a lot of heartache. The advice is not scientific. It is not strictly legal. It is really just common sense. But how much better to consider such matters before you embark on your studies with all that is entailed in terms of long-term commitment and financial hardship.

Before doing that you should understand a little about the functions of the GMC.

The General Medical Council

The GMC must be distinguished from the medical trade association, the British Medical Association (BMA) and from the Royal Colleges, which have distinct responsibilities for those practising within their specialty.

Whatever the changes effected as a result of the White Paper, the GMC will retain its core role in relation to the keeping and maintenance of the Medical Register and the Specialist Registers including the GP Register. It is important to grasp that the GMC is concerned with registration status and not with employment or contractual issues between doctors and employers.

The Medical Register exists to ensure that only those currently regarded as fit to practise may describe themselves as "registered medical practitioners" and provide medical advice and treatment to patients. In an effort to enhance the protection afforded by the Register, the CMO recommended, and the White Paper endorses, that a system of "recorded concerns" should be implemented. All concerns would be recorded on the Register thereby alerting employers and the public and these would be reviewed regularly by a national body.

Medical schools are now required to have Fitness to Practise procedures but of particular interest to those of you entering medical school in the next few years is a scheme already mooted by the GMC and now recommended by the CMO. The proposal is that medical students would be awarded "student registration" with a GMC "affiliate" operating fitness to practise systems within medical schools in parallel with those in place for registered doctors. Research has been emerging for some time that a student who behaves irresponsibly at medical school, or who regularly performs poorly in examinations, or who demonstrates a diminished capacity for self-improvement may well be the one who is likely to run into problems at a later stage. On 15 January 2007 the GMC and the Council of Heads of Medical Schools (CHMS) issued draft guidance on student fitness to practise.

The GMC currently has important functions in relation to medical education and qualifications. The CMO recommended that the role of the GMC to set the content of the medical undergraduate curriculum and to inspect and approve medical schools should be transferred to a body currently known as the Postgraduate Medical Education and Training Board (the PGETB). Given the GMC's role in creating and maintaining a clear and unambiguous set of standards for medical practice (incorporated into Good Medical Practice) and its responsibility for setting overarching principles and even for defining what is meant by a "good doctor", it was difficult to see the justification for change or how the system would work. The White Paper now recognises that there are benefits from having a single body overseeing medical education but seeks to preserve the expertise of the organisations currently undertaking this role. It endorses the model favoured by the GMC with the GMC overseeing undergraduate education and continuing professional development and the PGETB continuing to oversee postgraduate education. This scheme will be reviewed in 2011.

Whereas the bulk of complaints are dealt with at a local level, I shall concentrate in this chapter on regulation as currently exercised by the GMC since it is that process which may bring your registration into question and could even lead to the erasure of your name from the Medical Register. Over the past few years a great deal of attention has focused on the regulatory function of the GMC but it seems that further changes are now on the way.

First, it is useful to have a short historical overview of what has happened over the last three decades. The media has often portrayed the GMC as only being interested in sex and indecency and in the 1970s there was a vestige of truth in that the regulatory jurisdiction of the GMC, other than for health issues and convictions, was limited by statute to cases involving *serious* professional misconduct. Complaints about clinical matters were mainly concerned with general practitioners who failed to visit their patients or who failed to refer them to hospital. It is a reflection of the times that by the 1980s there had been a marked shift towards complaints of a clinical nature involving both GPs and hospital doctors and, correspondingly, an increasing focus on patient safety.

A number of cases also raised difficult ethical issues, for instance, the selling of kidneys for transplantation (the Turkish Kidney case), aspects of complementary medicine, female circumcision and cases about the ending of life. Irresponsible prescribing of drugs has been a topical subject for some years and allegations of dishonesty have featured all too often. Those complaints frequently arose in the context of clinical drug trials or research, the dishonest completion of CV's, dishonest claims for home visits or the giving of misleading evidence. All of these cases used to fall under the umbrella of an allegation of serious professional misconduct and the disciplinary arm of the GMC.

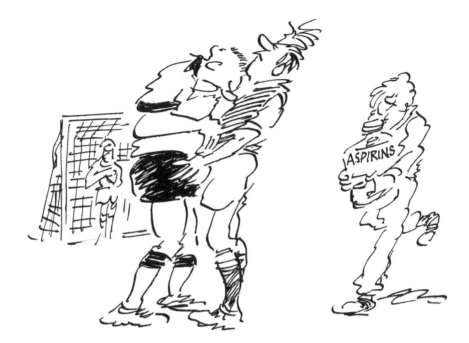

Then there were health cases in which a doctor's health was believed to be seriously impaired (usually in the context of drug or alcohol abuse or mental health problems) and in the main those cases which reached a hearing before the Health Committee involved doctors who lacked insight and would not accept voluntary restrictions upon their practice. The only remaining category of cases was those in which a doctor's fitness to practise was called into question as a result of a criminal conviction.

Then in 1995, in response to public pressure and to the concern of the GMC itself to have this power, the Medical (Professional Performance) Act was passed enabling the GMC for the first time to deal with poorly performing doctors. The Performance Procedures added an additional tool to the armoury and filled a gaping hole through which many inadequate doctors had slipped over the years. However, the importance of these procedures has been diminished by further changes.

Yet more reform was demanded, and this led the GMC to undertake an extensive overhaul of its constitution and procedures. The Medical Act 1983 (Amendment) Order 2002 substantially changed the way in which the profession was to be regulated by introducing a new test which involves answering the question "Is this doctor's fitness to practise impaired?" Section 35C Medical Act 1983 as amended provides that a person's fitness to practise may be regarded as "impaired" by reason of misconduct, deficient professional performance (including competence), a conviction or caution in the UK or elsewhere, adverse physical or mental health or by reason of the determination of a regulatory body in the UK or elsewhere.

In passing, it is right to highlight that the GMC has jurisdiction over UK registered doctors who are convicted of criminal offences abroad or who are disciplined by a foreign regulatory body just as it has jurisdiction over UK registered doctors whose professional conduct falls short of the standards expected when practising abroad. So, a drunken brawl in Benidorm or unlawful sexual activity in Canada may well place your registration in doubt. That is the price paid for the privilege of being on the UK Medical Register.

Rules implementing the new framework came into force on 1 November 2004 and the scheme effectively amalgamated the old procedures into one set of fitness to practise procedures. The aim was to facilitate an holistic view of a doctor since experience suggests that poor performance, misconduct and ill health are often difficult to disentangle. It may be helpful to bear this in mind should you find yourself going through a sticky patch or should you see a friend or colleague floundering. Whatever the reason, patients deserve to be protected, and a sick or exhausted doctor is often an inadequate or dangerous doctor.

To date, it has been panels of the GMC which have adjudicated in cases where it is alleged that a doctor's fitness to practise has been impaired. But that system has come in for much criticism. Even though large numbers of lay members have been involved for many years and may even constitute the majority of an adjudicating panel, and even though members of the GMC itself no longer sit on the Fitness to Practise panels, there is a widely held perception that regulation is effected by doctors who are intent on protecting their own and that the GMC has shown that it is not capable of adequately protecting the public.

As well as seeking primary legislation to ensure that lay members outnumber professionals on the Council itself, the White Paper adopts the recommendations of the CMO who proposed that much more of the regulatory workload should be carried out at a local level by GMC affiliates with an Independent Tribunal (rather than GMC panels) adjudicating in the more serious fitness to practise cases. The GMC would, however, retain its powers to investigate and assess doctors. The hope is that this will increase the transparency and public accountability of judgements about a doctor's registration and thus enhance public confidence. There are many hurdles, including funding, to be overcome before any Independent Tribunal is established and the timescale is unclear. So watch this space as this too could be an interesting topic for discussion at interview.

Not only does it seem that the GMC will soon lose its adjudicatory functions but there have been changes in the appellate process. Over the last few years, Judges of the High Court rather than Law Lords sitting in the Privy Council have been hearing appeals concerning doctors. This has led to some variation in approach and a resulting lack of consistency which is unhelpful to both complainants and doctors. But a decision of the Court of Appeal in January 2007 has reaffirmed that Fitness to Practise panels are normally best equipped to deal with matters of sanction.

A further change in recent years acts as a control on the way matters are handled by the GMC but also contributes to the stress of being a doctor against whom a serious complaint is made. If a decision of the GMC panel is considered to be too favourable to a doctor, an appeal lies to the High Court at the instigation of a body now calling itself The Council for Healthcare Regulatory Excellence (CHRE) rather than its formal name, The Council for the Regulation of Health Care Professionals (CRHCP). It is now proposed that the GMC should also have a right of appeal where it considers that too lenient an approach has been adopted by one of the Fitness to Practise Panels.

Continuing professional development and revalidation

It had been the intention of the GMC to introduce revalidation every five years in April 2005, the aim being to ensure that a doctor remains fit to practise throughout his professional life. But the process envisaged by the GMC was heavily criticised by Dame Janet Smith as being inadequate and consequently the GMC announced that the implementation of revalidation was to be postponed "for the time being". The CMO recommended a process of "re-licensure" for all registered doctors and "re-certification" for those doctors on the Specialist or GP registers. His recommendations are adopted in the White Paper and the emphasis is now on a positive affirmation of the doctor's entitlement to practise and not simply the apparent absence of concerns. How this is to be effected is anything but clear and some of the proposals may run into the sands of EU law because any doctor qualified to practise in his/her own home member state is entitled as of right to practise in the UK. Practice in the UK cannot be made conditional upon some UK certification.

Whatever system is devised and eventually implemented, it is essential to grasp that you are embarking on a lifelong journey of continuing professional development and assessment in a demanding climate in which the safety of patients and your fitness to practise is the key. Regular appraisal of course already features prominently for every doctor young and old.

Provisional registration

Since August 2005 anyone graduating from medical school has had to undertake further general clinical training within a 2-year (F1 and F2) Foundation Programme (see Chapter 10). There has been some criticism of placements made under the Foundation Programme with some of the stars complaining that they have not been placed in Foundation Hospitals but perhaps concern should focus on those who really need close supervision in high quality units to ensure they meet the standards that the public deserves. During the programme you will be expected to take increasing responsibility for patients under the supervision of more experienced doctors. To enable you to carry out your duties, you will get provisional registration in F1 and section 15 Medical Act 1983, as amended, provides that you *"shall be deemed to be registered as a fully registered practitioner"*. Even if student registration is not introduced, you will at that point become subject to the Fitness to Practise procedures of the GMC and the GMC must be told about any risk to patients or the public posed by you.

Provisional registration with the GMC gives F1s (previously described as pre-registration house officers or PRHOs) the rights and privileges of a doctor. In return they must meet the standards of competence, care and conduct set by the GMC. In December 2004, the Education Committee of the GMC produced a radically revised version of *The New Doctor* which, when finally implemented by legislation, will require

New Doctors to demonstrate through assessment that they have achieved defined outcomes before they can be considered fit to become fully registered practitioners.

During the 2 years of your Foundation Programme you will also be expected to deepen your awareness of medico-legal and ethical issues and to understand and apply the duties of doctors under the law but be reassured that advice is available to you from a number of sources. So, faced with the prospect that you will all at some point in your career face a complaint, what can you do to prepare yourself for practice so as better to face the challenges?

Know the system and to whom to turn for advice

It may seem self-evident that, by the time you qualify, you should be well informed about the system within which you are going to work but will you be? It is not for a lawyer to try and guide you through the jungle of the NHS, but it is my experience that ignorance of the system is sometimes a factor in a complaint. A constant refrain is "I did not know who to turn to for advice" or "I did not understand that was how the system worked". You need to be aware that your university continues to play an important part in your

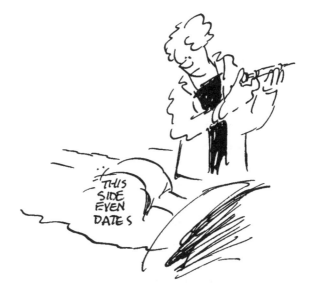

Foundation Programme and that you will have an educational supervisor. You may also have a mentor. You are still a doctor in training and as such you are required to be supervised. Others have the responsibility to do this and to provide you with continuing instruction.

At the time of writing, the process of selection for Specialist Training is under review and the future is uncertain for junior doctors but there will be others more senior (whatever they may be called in the future) to whom you can turn for advice and often you will need guidance from your consultant. You must not be reluctant to admit that you need a bit of help or advice or that you would prefer to see someone else insert a central line again before you try on your own. Of course, you do not want to be the person who always says no, but there is nothing wrong with expressing a wish to learn through experience and with requesting relevant instruction and supervision. A degree of humility may avert a disaster. Arrogance is a recipe for disaster.

If you have concerns about the health or behaviour of a colleague you should be aware that there are organisations which support sick doctors. You have a professional responsibility to take action if you believe that patients may be at risk of harm from another doctor's or healthcare professional's conduct, performance or health, including problems arising from alcohol or substance abuse. You need to understand the role of hospital managers and you need to know what services the BMA can provide.

Medical defence organisations and insurance

You need to consider seriously becoming a member of one of the medical defence organisations which many people think are only concerned with insurance. You may ask why if you are a student or are employed within a National Health Service hospital and therefore covered against claims under Crown Indemnity. The answer is that you will not be covered under the National Health Service Litigation Authority (NHSLA) or other schemes if you are in general or private practice. Furthermore, you will not be covered by your employer's scheme for legal representation should you face a complaint whether at local or GMC level or should you need to attend an inquest and require separate representation. You may even need advice as to whether you should be insisting on separate representation.

If you are undertaking locum jobs, you should always be very careful to check the position as to insurance. Locums are particularly vulnerable since they are not always given adequate induction into the unit in which they are working and because many locum appointments are very short and other healthcare professionals may not know the limits of the locum's competence. The quality of locums varies enormously; some may be inexperienced trainees filling in time before obtaining a place on a formal training scheme, others will be doctors who either prefer the itinerant lifestyle or who need the flexibility because of other responsibilities. Some will be excellent but others may not have been able to obtain or keep long-term appointments and they are often the ones who feature in complaints.

But there are other very good reasons to join a defence organisation and keep up your membership. They provide an excellent service in terms of giving medico-legal advice through the dark and lonely hours of the night when you may be feeling unsupported not to mention exhausted. Such advice should not be undervalued. You may need someone on whom to vent your spleen at having been left exposed and want confirmation that you should be waking up a rather grumpy consultant or there may be a real problem which you need to talk through with someone, for instance as to the capacity of a patient to consent to treatment.

The MPS provides excellent and concise guides some of which are specifically directed at students and these are available on line even to non-members (www.mps.org.uk). The other organisations tend to reserve their guidance to members.

GMC publications

Since 1995, the GMC has published an ever-increasing number of publications giving positive guidance to doctors. The topics covered reflect the changing world in which you will be practising. Following the Shipman Inquiry, the GMC set about preparing a radically revised version of the core guidance for medical practitioners. The new version of Good Medical Practice came into effect on 13 November 2006 and, whilst it certainly goes rather further than previous versions, it remains to be seen whether it commands universal approval in terms of setting explicit standards for practice as urged by Dame Janet Smith. This booklet (which can be accessed on line) is essential reading for every person at every stage of medical education, training and practice.

The Duties of a Doctor set out at the beginning of Good Medical Practice (see Appendix 3) identifies the foundation stones for practice that are built upon in the more detailed guidance. Do not learn the guidance by heart or churn it out like a mantra and be aware that it is not exhaustive as it has to retain flexibility to cater for advances in medical science and the ingenuity of doctors. You will not always find the answer to your problem and that is why you need to know who to turn to for advice.

Valuable information is contained within The New Doctor and there are booklets on The Early Years, Seeking Patients' Consent (November 1998 and a bit old), Confidentiality (April 2004), Research, Serious Communicable Diseases, Maintaining Good Medical Practice, Withholding and Withdrawing Life-prolonging Treatment (much debated) as well as guidance on topics such as conducting intimate examinations and chaperones and all of these are updated from time to time.

There is also guidance for those referring doctors to the GMC, for managers, teachers, and complainants and also for practitioners who face a complaint though that may not provide much solace.

Worryingly some doctors whose registration is on the line are not aware of the guidance offered by the GMC. It emerges that they have never read it let alone thought about its implications upon their practice. Floundering under (gentle) cross-examination they say that they must have lost the booklet when they last moved house. With the advent of the Internet and the GMC website (www.gmc-uk.org) these excuses will not impress! Do not wait until you have a complaint or a problem; make a habit of reading and thinking about the guidance throughout your professional life and of consulting the GMC website on a regular basis. That is all part of continuing professional development and reflective learning.

Do not bury your head in the sand

For even the most experienced doctor receiving a letter from the GMC advising that a complaint has been received about the management of a patient or about your conduct or health is a traumatic experience however confident you may feel about the way you handled a patient or behaved.

Whether your reaction is one of sadness, disbelief or anger, remember that it is vital to address the matter promptly. Do not bury your head in the sand and hope it will go away; it won't and inaction is a recipe for disaster. All complaints deserve to be addressed promptly, courteously and carefully

Since May 2004, if the GMC receives a complaint or is notified of a conviction involving a custodial sentence, it will discuss the complaint with your employer at an early stage in order to ascertain whether there have been other concerns about your practice and to ensure that the GMC is not approaching a wider problem piecemeal. So, although this is a sensitive area and you may be loathe to broadcast the fact you have been the subject of a complaint, it will always be wise to tell an appropriate person about it straight away. It may be helpful to get your oar in first and hopefully help and support will be offered to you.

At the earliest opportunity contact your defence organisation and start putting your tackle in order. Many a doctor (both young and experienced) could have been saved the ordeal of a protracted investigation or a full hearing if she/he had taken this course and received and accepted measured medico-legal advice at an early stage.

You may think that you are in the best position to know whether you got it seriously wrong or whether your fitness to practise is impaired, but almost certainly you are not! You are unlikely to be totally objective, you may be inexperienced and you cannot be expected to have a full grasp of the legal position. You need to be realistic and to think constructively. A full explanation may result in complete exculpation or it may reveal that you need some further training or help. Your clinical reasoning may not be clear from your notes or maybe the patient simply misunderstood what you were trying to say. Perhaps you documented the conversation in the medical notes or made a private record for your own purposes. An expert opinion may be needed or it may be necessary to take prompt steps to identify and take statements from others (perhaps a receptionist, a nurse or a practice manager) who may have overheard a conversation or taken a telephone call but who may in time move away.

You need to bear in mind that any letter written on your behalf should accurately reflect your case. Lawyers have an unfortunate habit of exposing any discrepancy between the case advanced and an earlier letter written by the advisers and it will not impress if you respond that you did not bother to check that the response reflected your case. Meticulous preparation undoubtedly pays off at every stage.

Strict time limits may apply so it is important that you give your advisers the maximum amount of time to investigate your case and draft a response. They will not be able to do your case justice if you have delayed until 24 hours before the deadline.

Professionalism and complaints

The real key to avoiding the pitfalls (and therefore the lawyers) lies in adopting a thoroughly professional approach. Apart from protecting patients, one of the purposes of regulation is to promote professionalism and any standards should incorporate the concept of professionalism which it is recommended should be placed in the contracts of all doctors.

Interestingly, in explaining what Good Medical Practice is about, the 2006 version of the guidance says, *"Good Medical Practice sets out the principles on which good medical practice is founded; these principles together describe medical professionalism in action."*

Surveys about what patients want of their doctors reflect the definition of a Good Doctor quoted at the beginning of this Chapter but also stress the importance of effective communication both oral and written. As patients' groups achieve a louder voice and mediation becomes more commonplace, it is apparent that many patients welcome the opportunity to come face to face with the doctor. This requires courage, an ability to listen and respond appropriately as well as sensitivity. It may be difficult but it is surprising how even strong views soften in this situation.

Saying sorry

It is always worthwhile stepping back and asking why patients complain? Research suggests that the great majority want an apology, explanation or inquiry; some want help coping; an even smaller percentage seek financial compensation and just a few favour disciplinary action. It is my experience that patients and their families are usually extraordinarily forgiving and understanding. They rarely want to see a doctor (particularly a young and inexperienced one) struck off. They want to discover what went wrong and why. They want to be reassured that others will not suffer the same fate and that there has not been an institutional or systems failure. So often it becomes clear that the "error" is not that of one individual but a pattern of complex interwoven problems. By asking awkward questions, a patient often reveals flaws in the system or that the premises or equipment are inadequate. An important quality in a doctor is an ability to listen quietly and also to accept constructive criticism when it is warranted.

Unfortunately, much of our legal system tends to confuse and obfuscate the issues of importance to patients by denying them the information they really want. Inquiries, if properly handled, may serve a useful purpose but not if they are conducted like witch-hunts or in an unnecessarily adversarial style. But why let it get that far? How much better to address the needs of the patient at the bedside or at least as soon as practicable after the mishap and thereby avoid the need for a complaint altogether.

In one memorable case in which a doctor had given false information to the brother of a deceased patient, the brother broke down after the doctor had been found guilty of serious professional misconduct (the test applied in conduct cases before November 2004) and erased from the Register and pleaded that he did not want that result. All he had wanted was to ascertain what investigations the doctor had undertaken but, as he said, once the doctor had lied, he had no option but to make a complaint. The moral of that tale is simple.

How often does one hear the cry "Why has it taken 3 years for us to hear the doctor say he is sorry?" Not infrequently it is an expert witness who says to the patient or relative "I am so sorry that the system let you down" or "I am so sorry that we doctors were not able to achieve a better outcome for you".

Happily it is now well recognised that it is both acceptable and indeed crucially important for a doctor to be able to say he is sorry that he was not able to achieve a better outcome for a patient and that he would be happy to sit down and explain what happened at a time convenient to the patient or relatives. Wise doctors frequently avert complaints by adopting this course and I hope they pass this lesson on. This advice is now encapsulated in Good Medical Practice at Paragraphs 30–31.

It is, of course, important not to rush into an apology or explanation in a moment of panic. As a junior doctor you will need advice from your seniors and very likely from your defence organisation and it is important to

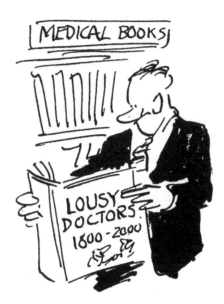

differentiate between an expression of regret coupled with an explanation (which is nearly always appropriate) and an acknowledgement of fault which may sometimes be called for but only after advice has been received.

Honesty and integrity

The doctor–patient relationship should be a partnership designed to achieve the best outcome for a patient. Honesty and integrity are fundamental to this relationship. Patients entrust doctors with their health and well-being and most complaints result from a breakdown in the professional relationship due to a loss of trust. Patients, their relatives, and members of the public are entitled to rely on the word of a doctor. Most people would agree with the view expressed by the Privy Council some years ago that "there is no room for dishonest doctors within the profession". Dishonesty in personal life may lead to criminal proceedings and a conviction. The short message is that dishonesty in any sphere of your life may impair your fitness to practise even if it has no connection with your professional life. Honesty should pervade all aspects of your dealings with patients, your paperwork, the certificates you complete, claims that you make for expenses and requests for study leave and the way you manage your own financial affairs.

Honesty is also of prime importance in the conduct of research as many doctors have learned to their cost. False data, fictitious claims in research papers or sloppily conducted research or clinical drugs trials may place patients at risk and bring reputable institutions into disrepute whilst discouraging members of the public from participating in valuable research. Moreover, the truth will usually emerge. It is possible to track entries through computers and it will usually become apparent if you use your own blood, urine, and electrocardiogram (ECG) trace to provide the data or if you have used a colleague's password to alter records. Some doctors are regrettably prepared to go to great lengths to earn a modest fee from a pharmaceutical company or to obtain a job for which they are inadequately equipped and that is a sure recipe for disaster on many counts.

Even in the early years you may be required to attend to give evidence, perhaps at an Inquest. There is no room for gilding the lily on oath. Giving misleading evidence is seriously regarded. If you are faced with an awkward encounter with a family member in the corridor in accident and emergency (A and E), it may be fruitful to try and think through the consequences of an ill-judged comment or perhaps a kindly white lie. A communications workshop threw up a perfect example: a young doctor is faced with the unenviable task of conveying to a distraught father in A and E that his child has been killed in a car accident. She knew that it had not been possible to control the child's pain but when asked by the father for reassurance that the child had suffered no pain, she said (wholly understandably and very kindly) that the child had been unconscious from the time she arrived at hospital. Is that acceptable?

There can be little doubt but that the student gave the humane response but may such an answer lead to problems? An Inquest will take place. The young doctor attends and gives the same evidence but it emerges that in fact the child was fully conscious on admission and was screaming uncontrollably. The doctor's otherwise entirely proper evidence may well be undermined. The coroner may smell a rat and consequently refer the case to the GMC for an inquiry. Without in any way underestimating the awful dilemma faced by the doctor caught on the hop, would it not have been better to try and find some way of avoiding answering the father's question without telling an untruth?

Unfortunately, dishonesty or a lack of candour is a frequent cause of complaints. Such complaints can be avoided.

Effective communication

Oral communication

Bad communication is probably the biggest single cause of complaints and it is closely linked to the topic of honesty. Unlike previous generations, today's doctors have had extensive instruction in communication skills but it is a feature of the system that it is often the greenest shoots who are the most exposed whether in A and E or as the house officer clerking in a patient. There is a world of difference between acting out how you would deal with a particular situation in a workshop and having to face the cold reality of telling a patient that he has cancer. Such news may be greeted with silence, anger, disbelief or by a flood of questions to which you may well not know the answer.

All doctors, at whatever stage of their professional lives, need to have a plan which enables them to extricate themselves from tricky situations whether in terms of concluding a conversation, creating an opportunity to take advice or just giving them additional time. Patients are usually understanding of the young doctor who says that he needs to speak to someone senior or who admits he does not know the answer or that the team does not yet have all the information it needs to answer the question. But the query must be followed through and the answer conveyed reasonably promptly. A brash or confrontational approach may easily lead to a complaint.

By its nature, medical practice is rarely predictable. You will inevitably be confronted by difficult situations, which require quick thinking. You need to develop a habit of logical and rational problem solving. Certain ethical tools to which you will be introduced may help you in this process. You may encounter a patient who has decided to conduct a lie down protest at your feet until you meet his demands and who, when you ask the porters to move him, then says "I have got a back problem, don't touch me or I shall sue the hospital and have you charged with assault". In general practice an abusive and aggressive drug addict may come into the surgery when you are alone in the premises at night and demand a prescription. And then there is the anxious relative who pleads with you for information about a patient to whom you have not been able to speak about sharing confidential material. Or, if you are a woman, you may be faced with a man who comes in and demands to see a "doctor" or a "real doctor". Sometimes you will need to think very fast and you must always be able to justify your actions.

There is a common maxim that, if you listen to the patient, he will give you the diagnosis. That is plainly over-simplistic but an analysis of complaints does reveal that so often clues are to be picked up if not in the verbal language of the patient or carer then from their body language or from what the patient does not say. Silence speaks volumes and hence the advice that you will receive throughout your training not to be afraid of silences. Some of the most important information emerges at those times.

In terms of effective communication and avoiding complaints, an awareness of cultural, social, and educational factors is clearly important. One mother may telephone the out of hours service very diffidently but describing with remarkable accuracy the signs and symptoms of meningitis. She concludes by apologising profusely for calling the doctor at night and for fussing unnecessarily. Another may be a constant caller whom it may be tempting to dismiss as a nuisance. You will need to be on the alert for such situations and you must be mindful of the potential for disaster if you dismiss the second mother's concerns. But even lawyers understand that resources are not infinite and that doctors have to make uncomfortable decisions about priorities every day of the week.

Situations like this not infrequently found complaints. What can you do to avoid them? In making a few suggestions, I rely on examples drawn from real cases. Although the information passed to you by the message service or the receptionist will be very important, you need to try to speak to the persons concerned yourself. The patient himself may know, for instance, that Dengue Fever was prevalent in the particular area he visited. He may be able to give you a more accurate picture than his anxious mother. Try to avoid the information being passed to you second hand if the patient is able to speak to you directly. Elicit as much history and background as you can to establish whether the history given to the message service is accurate or whether it has been accurately recorded. This may enable you to form a view as to whether the patient lost consciousness and if so, whether this was a simple faint. Ensure that the message you were passed is appended to the notes. Make a very careful record of your contact with the patient so that others who take over the care of the patient can see how matters have developed and always date and time your record. If you are left in any doubt about the urgency of the situation, visit or arrange for someone else to do so in order that a proper assessment can be made. So much of medicine involves weighing up the risks and to do this properly you need information.

You may well not be able to make a firm diagnosis but if you fail to make an assessment on the basis of a proper history and examination if called for, you will be an easy target for the lawyers. Provided you can show that you have followed the proper process, even if you have made an error of judgement, your fitness to practise on the grounds of misconduct or deficient performance may be beyond reproach.

That effective communication is so important is illustrated by a complaint in the early 1990s against a doctor who was called to see a baby in North Harrow. After several calls he visited somewhat reluctantly. The baby was moribund and covered in a rash. The mother was distraught but tried her best to communicate her anxiety to the doctor telling him that the rash had persisted even after she had pressed a tooth mug against the baby's skin. The doctor was entirely dismissive of the mother's concerns and left. At the hearing he even insisted that there was no need to get the baby to hospital as it was just "smallpox". You can probably guess the rest – the baby had fulminating meningococcal septicaemia and died shortly afterwards. The doctor had resolutely failed to listen and had failed to pick up any of the cues. Just because you have acquired considerable scientific expertise do not forget that common sense and common humanity remain vital tools for a doctor.

It is common experience that people only retain small parts of the information they are given particularly if they are being given bad news or technical information such as may need to be conveyed when you are seeking consent. From a lawyer's perspective and for your own protection, it can be very helpful to offer the patient the opportunity to have a friend or relative present. This may have the added advantage of getting over tricky problems about confidentiality in a case where an anxious relative wants to know the diagnosis or the prognosis or about the risks of surgery, provided of course, that the patient agrees to the information being shared. But be scrupulously careful and sensitive about matters that the patient does not wish to share.

Having a member of the nursing staff present can have advantages too. For one, you will be able to explain to the patient that if he has a query, the nurse may be able to reinforce what you have said or help in other ways and that if she cannot, she will be able to pass on any concerns to the medical team. From a forensic point of view, the presence of another person may also be helpful in terms of showing that you did, for example, discuss other treatment options or explain the risks. In order that your witness can later be tracked down through Human Resources, identify them in your note. Months or years later when your rotation has taken you to fresh pastures it will be very difficult to remember who was there and you may therefore lose a valuable supporting witness.

If you listen to your patient (and his carers) and check his understanding of what you have said, you will avoid the two major pitfalls that found complaints.

Written records

Just as important as effective oral communication is the keeping of good written records. Lawyers are very boring about this but time and time again, complaints could have been avoided or disputes cleared up more easily if there had been a clear, accurate, and contemporaneous record, legibly written and clearly timed, dated and signed. Many young doctors complain that they have graduated from medical school without having had to write a discharge summary, a referral letter or having learned how to complete a death certificate. But, that cannot excuse bad ones. The writing of records and completion of forms are skills that have to be learned and practised.

Even lawyers appreciate that there are times when, because of the pressure of an emergency, it is only possible to make a short contemporaneous note recording the most salient points. That is not to say that there is anything wrong in writing a retrospective note provided it is clear that is what it is and the note is clearly marked as such. Indeed retrospective notes can be extremely useful in all forms of litigation. Examples might include a fuller note made by way of elaboration after an anaesthetic disaster when the pressure is off and when perhaps it is noted that a particular drug has been inadvertently omitted from the drug chart. A retrospective note which explains more fully the sequence of events or the clinical reasoning behind a decision will often assist in understanding why a particular course has been adopted. After a difficult telephone call from a patient or after an encounter with an aggressive or abusive patient, a carefully written retrospective note may save the day. But keep any note factual and do not be tempted to speculate or rationalise with the benefit of hindsight.

Inaccurate or incomplete drug charts or certificates completed without reading the form or without seeing and assessing the patient provide easy targets for the lawyers. Whatever the temptation, never be tempted to embellish or exaggerate and do not expect any mercy if you alter or tamper with records of any sort. By putting your name to a piece of paper or making an entry in the computer records you are saying, "Believe me, I am a doctor and this is accurate and true". Patients and the authorities are entitled to rely on your word whether you are certifying a passport application, a form seeking benefits or simply making a record in the notes.

Referral letters are a common source of complaint. A complaint may emanate from the Consultant to whom you have made the referral because the letter contains no useful information and therefore denies the Consultant the opportunity to assess the urgency of the case with the result that Mrs X is not given an urgent appointment because you have failed to note that, in addition to a breast lump, she has a bleeding nipple. Patients sometimes have good cause for complaint because of derogatory language or inaccuracies in the history given. On any basis it is good medicine and good practice to write proper informative letters and offensive or sarcastic letters do nothing for the doctor–patient relationship. Tact and sensitivity are essential qualities for all doctors particularly since some patients will now choose to see their medical records.

Communications with colleagues and other health professionals

A third aspect of effective communication relates to communication with medical colleagues and other health professionals. Increasingly doctors work in multi disciplinary teams and members of the team will have different spheres of expertise but co-operation and discussion is essential. Good doctoring requires considerable man management skills not only in terms of delivering good care to patients but also in terms of dealing with medical colleagues, managers and other health professionals. Not all are charming, modest and easy-going individuals but it is that diversity that makes medicine so interesting.

Respect for the contribution of others is vital; a lack of mutual respect is a frequent cause of complaints and the labour ward provides a steady flow of work for the lawyers because, understandably, experienced midwives sometimes think that they have greater experience than a junior doctor making a rare foray into the labour ward in the course of a short rotation. But respect needs to be tempered with caution as ultimately a patient's care will normally be the responsibility of the doctor. Sometimes questions need to be asked and you have to be prepared to stand your ground.

A GMC case in 1993 represented a watershed in this area, highlighting the importance of effective communication within a team. A doctor who had for years led an itinerant life working as a locum anaesthetist was found guilty of serious professional misconduct as a result of his grossly incompetent management of a patient undergoing major surgery under general anaesthesia. Before this incident, a number of nurses and operating department assistants had become seriously worried about his behaviour. They had alerted the Head of Department to their concerns telling him that the anaesthetist used to eat sandwiches and read *The Daily Telegraph* during procedures. The Head of Department failed to investigate or act upon those concerns. A complaint was made to the GMC and subsequently he was found guilty of serious professional misconduct. Two lessons are to be learned from this case: first and foremost, a Head of Department or a doctor working in a similar role has a direct responsibility for patients in his department's care and, secondly, there must be effective communication between all members of the healthcare team as well as with patients and relatives. Under the new test his fitness to practise would surely be regarded as impaired on the ground of either misconduct or deficient professional performance. The safety of patients was at stake.

A more recent illustration of this point is to be found in the Bristol paediatric cardiac surgery case. At the heart of the case against Dr Roylance (the Chief Executive but nevertheless a registered medical practitioner) was the allegation, ultimately found proved, that he had failed to listen to the concerns voiced to him, failed to heed numerous warnings, failed to investigate and thereby failed to safeguard the interests of the babies undergoing surgery in his hospital. He was found guilty of serious professional misconduct and erased. Much the same complaint was found proved against Mr Wisheart, the Senior Surgeon and Medical Director, who was also erased.

A further example of the importance of communicating effectively with nurses and carers involved a decision by a general practitioner to withdraw feeding from an elderly stroke patient who resided in a nursing home for which he was responsible. There were undoubtedly two points of view about her condition both worthy of consideration. The general practitioner chose not to consult with the health professionals in the home. He simply issued an instruction that feeding should be discontinued, to the great distress of some of the team who had cared for the patient over a number of years. That was his downfall. Had he discussed the matter with the staff he would have been made aware that there was a difference of opinion about the patient's ability to swallow and about her overall condition. He would not have incurred the wrath of the nurses and carers and most importantly, he would have learned relevant information which might or might not have caused him to make a different decision. One thing is pretty certain: had he communicated better, he would probably not have faced a complaint.

Consent

This book does not purport to teach you medical law. Neither does this Chapter presume to give you advice about the process of seeking consent from a patient nor as to whether it is appropriate for you be involved in that process at all in your very early years. What it does seek to do is to alert you to the fact that lack of consent forms the basis of many complaints and hence it is a subject which deserves very serious consideration. Consent is a subject which is absolutely central to the trust patients are entitled to place in doctors. It is relevant from the very first day you go onto the wards or into a home or practice as a medical student. Patients are entitled to know who and what you are before they agree to confide in you or let you take a history or examine them.

Consent provides a defence to an allegation of assault or more accurately battery. Consent does not provide a doctor with a defence to negligent treatment or advice. The need for consent derives from the law's respect for the patient's right to decide. It provides a defence to an allegation of assault provided that the touching goes no further than is necessary for proper medical purposes. Be wary of the relative who purports to consent on the patient's behalf even if his views may help you make your own assessment as to what your unconscious patient might have wanted.

You should be entirely open that you are a medical student and indeed a senior doctor who wishes you to examine a patient or to perform some procedure should ensure he has the prior consent of that patient. There are very many reports of students being asked to intubate a patient or conduct some sort of examination on an anaesthetised patient and this is entirely unacceptable unless prior consent has been obtained. Do not be afraid to ask your senior whether consent has been obtained in advance for you to do this and, unless you receive a satisfactory answer, be prepared to say no. Pass on your concerns and you will have no problem in justifying your refusal.

Well-publicised cases on lack of consent concern the removal of the left leg when it was intended to remove the right and ovaries removed without consent in the course of a hysterectomy. But there are more subtle examples such as the touching of a woman's breasts without proper explanation; behaviour which, in turn, sometimes leads to an allegation of indecency.

You will in due course be thoroughly drilled in the necessity of completing hospital consent forms and far be it from me to detract from that practice. But it is worth being aware that consent does not have to be in writing. The importance of a consent form lies in the fact that it provides some evidence of what was said. It is, however, the quality and actual content of what was agreed that is of real importance. It follows that a good record of what was said and agreed, identifying who else was present and recording the salient points, will not only assist you should things go wrong but will also assist others involved in the patient's care in knowing what information was actually conveyed to the patient.

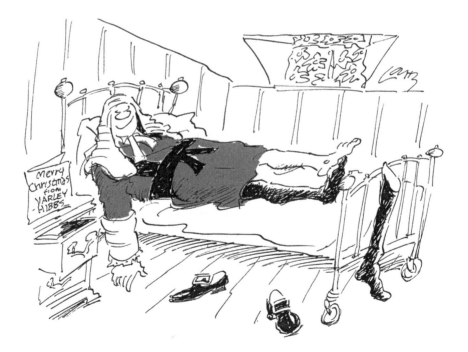

To be valid, consent must be given voluntarily by a person who is legally competent to give it. It must be preceded by proper information about the risks and benefits to enable the patient to give what is often called "informed consent". Assessment of capacity is not always straightforward and sometimes you will need to call on others to assist in this task. You should have regard to The Mental Capacity Act 2005 part of which became law on 1 April 2007 with the remainder due to be implemented on 1 October 2007.

The question of how much a patient must or should be told is often a vexed one. A balance has to be struck between the patient's entitlement to know matters which may affect his choice and not creating unnecessary fear. The patient is always entitled to be told the truth and to be given the information that he seeks or needs to have in a kind and straightforward way using clear language and drawings if they would assist.

It is vital to establish that the patient has understood what he is being told. Never shy away from checking this and asking whether a patient has any other queries. It is frequently these questions which reveal that the patient has misunderstood what is being proposed or alert you to his fears which can then be addressed.

Whilst the risk of injury to a nerve in the index finger may not be a decisive factor in the case of a professional singer considering hand surgery, the same risk may be unacceptable to a concert pianist or a surgeon. So, it will always be important to gauge what a patient hopes to achieve and what he fears. Your own views, whilst perhaps a helpful guide, cannot be regarded as decisive. Some patients do not want to know what you would do. Others may find that helpful.

It would be possible to recount innumerable cautionary tales relating to the seeking (so often inappropriately described as the 'taking') of consent which would serve to illustrate that this is a huge topic, which will confront and sometimes perplex you throughout your career. With experience, observation and study you will acquire a deeper understanding of the medico-legal and ethical issues involved.

That there are so many complaints alleging lack of consent underlines the importance of effective communication. It also highlights the importance of respecting the views of patients and their entitlement to be involved in decisions about their future care. A number of complaints arise out of well-meaning decisions: an example is a decision to proceed to an oophorectomy during a hysterectomy because of some abnormal findings even though specific consent has not been obtained. Doctors have no right to overrule the informed decisions of patients nor are they entitled to make assumptions about patients' wishes no matter how well intentioned their actions may be.

Consent is not a subject reserved to the operating theatre. Many GPs have found themselves at the wrong end of an allegation of indecent assault just because they have not thought fit to say to a woman whose chest they are listening to "Do you mind if I now check your breasts?" So easy and so effective, yet so often overlooked! Yet again one comes back to the need for a sensitive approach coupling kindness with proper professionalism and good manners.

In an emergency, do only the minimum required to save life or preserve the status quo thus leaving as many options as possible open until consent can be sought. You are very vulnerable if you do not lay the ground properly and in an emergency situation it is always essential to make good notes.

Confidentiality

Confidentiality is another complex subject and the finer points are way beyond the scope of this chapter. But here again it is central to the trust you must build up with your patients. The basic principle is simply stated. Patients have a right to expect that information about them will be held in confidence by their doctors and in general terms the obligation to maintain confidentiality persists even after a patient has died. If information is to be provided to others, there are procedures that must be followed. You will have read of concerns about the proposed NHS national database which would enable a large number of individuals to access confidential information. Whilst the sharing of information over the country may benefit patients in many ways, there are obvious anxieties that this may be contrary to the wishes of a patient or that the information may get in to the wrong hands. Can you think of any possible solutions?

Careless chat at a party is not acceptable however impressed your friends may be to hear that you have been attending to a famous politician or pop star. Neither paper nor computer records should be left where they can be seen by others. More than one doctor has got himself into trouble that way.

You should endeavour to ensure that your screen is positioned so that a patient cannot read about another patient on your computer.

You should note that there are circumstances in which disclosure of information is required by law: for instance in response to a court order or to satisfy a specific statutory requirement such as notification of a communicable disease. Information may need to be disclosed to those involved in the care of a patient requiring emergency treatment who is not able to give consent at the time or it may need to be disclosed in the public interest. Where a patient has refused consent and where there is a serious risk to the patient or others, disclosure may nevertheless be justified but it will be necessary for you to consider carefully whether the benefits to an individual (for instance the partner of someone suffering with HIV) or to society outweigh the interests of the patient in keeping the information confidential.

It follows that you must always be able to justify disclosure and you need to develop an awareness of those areas of the law that may give rise to a need for disclosure. These include child abuse, sex offenders, communicable diseases, providing information to a Coroner and certain other bodies, death certification, dealings with the Driver and Vehicle Licensing Agency (DVLA), and dealings with the GMC about a colleague whose fitness to practise may be impaired by alcohol, drugs or mental or physical illness. Each case needs to be considered on its own facts and provided you have followed the right procedures and asked yourself the right questions, you are unlikely to get into serious trouble. But I would suggest that, in your early years, this is an area in which it will usually be prudent to take advice from your seniors or your defence organisation.

Effective communication is a vital tool in dealing with questions of confidentiality and many potential problems can be overcome by commonsense coupled with imaginative handling. An important question in every case is "Does the patient have the capacity to consent to disclosure of confidential information?"

I have already touched upon the potential advantages of involving a relative or friend in certain discussions with the agreement of the patient and this will often be the way of allowing the anxious relative to learn more about the diagnosis or prognosis. It is so easy to ask a patient whether he/she is content for someone else to be present during a consultation, but so often this simple precaution is over looked.

You need to be careful that any consent to disclosure is still current and that it covers information you are being asked for. It is not uncommon for a doctor to get a telephone call from a spouse. Most enquiries will be well meaning and genuine and because you feel pretty sure that the other spouse would have agreed, your instinct may be to tell all. But has it occurred to you that the couple may now be estranged or that the consent that you got to disclose information about the breast lump does not cover a wider disclosure? Such a situation may arise in connection with a request to be told the results of a pregnancy or blood test or an enquiry as to whether Mrs X told you that she regularly consumes half a bottle of whisky a night.

Difficulties also arise in relation to children. For years a child has come to see you with her mother. Then she comes on her own or appears anxious about her mother's presence. Just as it is essential to preserve the trust as between doctor and patient, it is important that the parent child relationship should not be jeopardised. Can you engineer a few minutes alone with the child in order to try to persuade her that it is in her interests that her mother should know the situation? Would she like you to speak to her mother alone first in order to break the ice? Does a question of abuse arise and can you justify non-disclosure to a statutory agency? Or do the interests of the child and her blank refusal to give consent to disclosure require that you maintain her confidentiality? You will have heard of the Gillick case involving contraceptive advice.

In terms of confidentiality there are many other areas that require careful thought. These include audit, research, the provision of medical reports to insurers and the publication of papers. Overall, you need to develop an awareness of the complexity of the subject so that you are in a position to recognise when you may be approaching tiger country.

Preparing to give evidence

The idea of giving evidence may seem rather tame after the trials and tribulations of your training and after the clinical problems you will encounter on the wards. You may also think that you are unlikely to be required to give evidence early in your career. Alas, that is not the case. It may be tempting to think you can do it without much preparation after a long period on duty and without having gone back to your records and having refreshed your memory from your statement and the correspondence. You may relish the idea of returning to amateur dramatics and of outsmarting a lawyer who, you think, knows nothing about medicine and will not have done his preparation. Beware, medico-legal work is now a very specialised area and lawyers working in the field may be more clued up than you would expect even if their knowledge of medicine is pretty superficial.

But I would suggest that the reality of giving evidence whether in your own defence or in a case in which your management of a patient is under scrutiny is very different. Most doctors report that it is highly stressful and nearly all wish that they had been better prepared. Many doctors who are faced with giving evidence in their own defence in response to a complaint are their own worst enemies but rest assured that lawyers are the worst witnesses of all!

Of course, it pays to do thorough preparation well in advance. Make sure you are properly represented if need be. If you are asked to attend an inquest, ask yourself and your seniors whether you are the right person to go. You may be required to give some factual evidence but you are still a doctor in training and as such you are working under supervision. You are certainly not qualified to give expert evidence nor should you allow yourself to be trapped into trying to do that.

Do not automatically assume that you and the Trust have identical interests. Take every opportunity to go and watch your seniors give evidence. You may be asked whilst doing a psychiatric post in F2 or whilst working as a GP Registrar to go and give evidence at a Mental Health Review Tribunal (MHRT). This should be the job of the Consultant or at least a senior person who understands about the statutory criteria but unfortunately this task often falls to junior doctors who are not really equipped to deal with the complex issues that arise. You need to be prepared to stand your ground and say that you do not have the necessary expertise to perform the role. Ask instead whether you may go as an observer so that you may learn from watching your senior.

If you are facing a complaint in which others are also implicated, consider carefully and in advance whether there may be a potential conflict of interest which should preclude you from being represented by the same person and be prepared to seek and take advice about this. You may not be the right person to judge whether or not a conflict could arise and Day 3 of a hearing will be too late.

You cannot start preparation an hour before the hearing. You may be giving evidence about events some months or years ago and a lot of water will have flowed under the bridge. You may need to see your solicitor or to have a conference with counsel. You certainly need to have your papers paginated and in the same form as your advisers and the tribunal or you will be forever rustling through reams of paper. Even if the lawyers or judge is trying to press you, you need to remember that you are in control of the tempo. Ensure that you understand the question. Do not be afraid to ask for the question to be repeated. Questions are not always clear and the thinking behind them may be muddled or plain wrong particularly if the subject is technical but remember that there is no excuse for discourtesy or being patronising.

Never be afraid to say that you cannot now remember or that you cannot answer the question. Do not fall in to the trap of thinking you can anticipate the questions or that you know where they are leading. Answer as concisely as you can but do not allow yourself to be pushed into giving a Yes or No answer just because of insistent questioning. Even experienced witnesses complain that they have felt pressurised into doing this when there was something else to be said by way of qualification and you have to be brave sometimes. Do not be afraid to say that you need time to find an entry in the nursing notes which weighed with you in making a particular decision. Do not be tempted to portray yourself as an expert when you are not. A quiet, calm, considered, and suitably modest approach is nearly always the best.

Concluding remarks

By now, some of you may be feeling that the climate is such that medicine is not for you. Experienced doctors may recognise some of the scenes I have described and be shuddering. But effective regulation is essential if the public is to be appropriately protected and confidence in the profession maintained. The fact that patients and the authorities are now readier to complain underlines the need to establish a partnership with patients and other health care professionals.

During the course of your professional life you may be subjected to harsh criticism. It will hurt but constructive criticism is to be valued and acted upon. Several doctors I have encountered could have avoided a GMC inquiry or even erasure had they been prepared to react positively or had they accepted well-meaning advice to consider another career path. Surgery or paediatrics may not be the right specialty for you to follow and even potentially good doctors may be square pegs in round holes. Many complaints reflect this and there are other areas with less patient contact in which you may excel.

There is no doubt that doctors are now under ever-increasing pressure and, although there has now been considerable reaction to the Shipman Report, the Report of the CMO and the White Paper, it is still too early to say how and when the system will be changed. Criticism of the profession, the training programmes and the system of regulation has been wide-ranging but my experience is that medical students do not feel overly discouraged. Some view the problems faced by the profession as a challenge to be met and undoubtedly the very great majority of doctors take their responsibilities to patients very seriously and put patient safety above all else. Most will not hesitate to take appropriate action if they believe that a colleague is putting patients at risk and most of us, in whatever profession, hope for a good friend who will tell us when things look as if they may be going wrong or when it is time to stop.

But, of course, there will be a few doctors who, for whatever reason, perform poorly or even plain badly. There will be some who act outside the limits of their competence. There may also still be some who do not have the courage to draw attention to a colleague's ill health or performance. And in any event, complaints will continue to be made and regrettably some are made maliciously or for reasons of internal politics. Many complaints can be avoided if you use your common sense and follow relatively simple guidance. Provided you approach the challenges that lie in wait – not just now but throughout your professional career – with a degree of humility and humanity, you have little to fear.

Dare I say that it is rarely the junior doctors freshly out of medical school and imbued (as the Shipman report concedes) with the new culture who fall into the traps I have identified. It is more frequently their seniors who are perhaps overwhelmed by paperwork and managerial duties or who are tired and burned out or who have forgotten some of the basic principles instilled during training. That leads me to hope that this chapter will be read not only by those considering a career in medicine but by medical students, those that teach and train them and indeed by doctors throughout their careers. I go further; it is possible that members of the public and the leaders of patients' groups will also find this book illuminating. Doctors, lawyers, and patients will all benefit if we can develop a greater understanding of each other and identify what makes a good doctor.

It is useful to remember that just as courts and legal procedure will be strange and perhaps uncomfortable for doctors, hospitals and medical jargon are pretty uncomfortable for most members of the public. Therein lies a lesson for both doctors and lawyers. We all need to communicate in a clear and effective way. We need to combine sensitivity and humanity with understanding. And of course, we should only act within the limits of our professional competence. Doctors need to earn and retain the confidence of their patients and to abide by the standards and principles of their profession. That is the best way of avoiding the pitfalls and the lawyers and of being a true professional.

REMEMBER

- Many complaints can be avoided by common sense.

- Keep abreast of new guidance

- In the event of a complaint, seek help and advice promptly from your medical defence organisation.

- Deal with complaints constructively and realistically.

- Learn from your mistakes and the mistakes of your colleagues.

- Medicine requires life long learning and reflection. It is a life choice.

- Heed career advice.

- Be prepared to say you are sorry.

- Try to understand your patients' viewpoint.

- Above all, listen to your patients and communicate with them effectively.

Postscript

On the decision to become a doctor rests the whole design and course of your life.

Being a doctor is something of a love–hate relationship. A recent graduate, who had more than her fair share of difficulties as a student, described the feeling like this: "I am now working in a friendly district general hospital and I love it. I love being a doctor – at least I hate some of it but I am glad I went through medical school, resits and all".

We also have had our doubts but are glad to be doctors or to have had the good fortune to work with the stars of the profession as well as with some who have sometimes not performed to the high standards patients are entitled to expect. Unlike the famous cricketer, WG Grace, who took 10 years to qualify as a doctor, and said: "Medicine is my hobby, cricket is my profession", we believe that professionalism should be central to the everyday life of all doctors. But doctors need diversions and we like the approach of Anton Checkov, who said "Medicine is my lawful wife and literature is my mistress. When I grow weary of one, I pass the night with the other. Neither suffers from my infidelity."

We cannot say what is right for you. We can only hope that we will have helped you towards your own well thought out decision. If you do decide that medicine is the career for you and are successful in gaining a place at medical school, we hope that "Learning Medicine" will be your friend and guide well into your professional career.

For the last words we turn first to Susan Spindler, original producer of the BBC documentary series *Doctors to Be*, who once thought of becoming a doctor but decided against:

Having observed hundreds of students and doctors over the past decade, I have a checklist of qualities I look for in my doctors. I should like you to be kind, clever, and competent. I want you to know your way around the system, both in hospital and in the community. I hope you will like and will empathise with your patients wherever humanly possible and fight to give them the best treatment. And I'd like to think that you'll have managed to hang on to some of the ideals which drew you to medicine in the first place.

And finally, to Dr Farhad Islam, who as a student contributed his impressions of his first delivery (p. 110) and recently showed so graphically in an article reproduced here by courtesy of the *British Medical Journal*, how the years of learning medicine come together to make a competent and humane doctor, not forgetting in a moment of drama the need to be the patient's friend.

This time it was not a drill*

The phone rang. It was ten past nine in the morning and I wasn't due to start work in the casualty department at St Mary's Hospital until the afternoon.

"Where are you? It's Dad here. There's been a major rail crash just down the road from you. Hundreds are injured."

I quickly changed and ran downstairs. I weaved in and out of the traffic on my bicycle, and within 2 minutes I was at the police cordon. I flashed my identity badge and was led to the scene of the disaster.

"Keep your bicycle helmet on, Doc. The paramedics are over there with some of the wounded."

One hour had passed since the fatal collision and already a slick rescue plan was in operation. There were five commuters lying on the ground, each white with fear, shivering, although it was not cold. They lay with charred or bloodied faces. Looking dazed and frightened, but all uncomplaining – happy just to be alive.

I approached the trauma triage coordinator.

"Hello, I'm a casualty officer. How can I help?"

I was directed to two wounded passengers yet to see a doctor. I felt as if I was on autopilot, driven by all the procedures that I had been taught and all the duty that had been ingrained in me. That feeling would continue for most of the day. Basics first – airway, breathing, circulation. I assessed a man with a blackened face. He was obviously in pain with a deformed broken lower right leg. A paramedic was squeezing a bag of fluid into his veins to prevent shock. It was soon emptied and we had to wait for the next fleet of ambulances for more bags. He was stabilised and put into an ambulance, all the while thanking those around him.

I caught sight of a woman on the ground being comforted by a friend. She was visibly shaking. I peered into a large gash in her forehead. We immobilised her spine and put her in an ambulance.

The coordinator told me that it was unlikely that anyone else would be brought out alive from the wreckage. It was time to go to Mary's now. I grabbed my bike and sped down the main road still feeling as if some kind of compelling force was driving me. The whole experience was just so surreal. I had read the major incident plan 2 years before and remember being impressed by the precision and detail. There would be a press room; one room would be set up as a mortuary. I was reminded of the mock simulations of major incidents in my student days. Then volunteer students had been daubed in make up blood to act as casualties.

The accident and emergency department was a hive of activity. What struck me was that there seemed to be order, there seemed to be a plan, and it was working. It quickly dawned on me why I had not been rung. Doctors from all departments and specialties had rushed to help.

I was allotted a patient to look after and immediately recognised her as the woman I had attended at the scene. Now, like all the other patients, she had a number and I would be responsible for her. Around every patient was a dedicated team of doctor plus nurse.

Never had I imagined a major incident running so efficiently, especially with the horrific severity of injuries. The major incident packs, used for the first time, had all the necessary forms. Medical students stood ready to rush blood samples to the laboratories. I glimpsed the sight of patients with major burns being whisked away for emergency surgery.

My duty was to stay with my patient to continually assess her condition, anticipate potential problems, investigate and repair her wounds and be her friend. She had a nasty head injury and remained pale and cold. My main concern after establishing that her airway, breathing, and circulation were stable was to recognise that she might have a skull fracture and underlying serious head injury. The appropriate monitoring and tests were done.

It is funny how little things impress on your mind – hearing about members of the public ringing to donate blood, the catering department sending down sandwiches and drinks for exhausted staff, the gratitude of patients. All the while I was with my team, other teams were treating their own patients. Some were dreadfully burned, others had fractured limbs, ruptured spleens, or head injuries. I stitched up my patient's wounds with the help of a medical student. The nurses dressed her other wounds and we transferred her to the adjoining ward.

Suddenly the department was quiet and then the debriefing – lots of emotion, satisfaction, and pride on all sides for the sheer professionalism shown not just by the medical and nursing staff but by the porters, receptionists, police, security, and caterers.

*Taken from *British Medical Journal* 1999; **319**: 1079.

Appendices

Appendix 1: Medical School Charter 2006

Part 1: The responsibilities of the medical student

Medical students undertake a degree in medicine with the aim of becoming medical practitioners. Whilst students do not yet have the full duties and responsibilities that go with being a registered medical practitioner, they are already in a privileged position with regards to patients and those close to them. In recognition of this, students must maintain a good standard of behaviour and show respect for others. By awarding a medical degree, a university is confirming that the graduate is fit to practise to the high standards that the GMC has set in its guidance to the medical profession, *Good Medical Practice*.

The GMC outlines the standards expected of a qualified doctor in *Good Medical Practice* and other guidance. Many of those standards apply to you as a medical student. Those of particular relevance are set out below:

1. The student will treat every patient politely and considerately.

As a student, you will:

1.1. treat each patient with respect.

1.2. make sure that the patient understands that you are a student and not a qualified doctor.

1.3. make sure the patient has agreed to your presence and involvement.

1.4. not continue interaction if the patient indicates a wish to stop.

1.5. dress in an appropriate professional manner that enables good communication with your patients.

1.6. acknowledge that patients have the right to expect that all health care workers and students should both appear and be professional.

During your training you will come into contact with many patients from a variety of backgrounds. Usually, your contact with patients will be for your benefit and not theirs. It is important that you approach each patient with respect. As a minimum, this means that you should make sure that patients understand that you are a student and that they have agreed to your presence and involvement with them. Be sensitive to their reactions and do not continue your interaction with them if they indicate that they have had enough.

Students as well as doctors must be prepared to respond to a patient's individual needs and take steps to anticipate and overcome any barriers to communication. In some situations this may require you to set aside your personal and cultural preferences in order to provide effective patient care.

Consideration for your patients affects how you choose to appear. Your dress and appearance should not interfere with your ability to communicate with your patients and their supporters. Fashion changes but patients have the right to expect that all health care workers and students appear professional. Dress which is too informal or is at the extremes of fashion may offend some patients. Good personal hygiene and grooming is essential.

Be aware that you are going to be in very close contact with patients. General appearance, facial expression and other non-verbal signals are important components of good communication in the wider UK community. Any form of dress which interferes with this (such as covering the face or wearing excessive jewellery) should be avoided.

2. The student will respect patients' dignity and privacy.

The student will:

2.1. address patients in professional way.

2.2. endeavour to preserve the patient's dignity at all times.

2.3. attempt to ensure the patient's privacy at all times.

Remember, patients are human beings not museum exhibits. Always ensure that the patient's dignity is preserved in the manner in which you address them. Err on the side of formality rather than familiarity unless the patient gives you specific permission to be more informal. Take care when examining a patient not to embarrass them by over-exposure. The level of acceptable exposure varies from individual to individual. Be aware of the wishes of your patient in this regard.

3. The student will listen to patients and respect their views.

It is easy to turn history taking into an interrogation, but a consultation is a two way process. Do not allow yourself to ignore what the patient has to say.

4. The student will respect and protect confidential information.

The student will not:

4.1. intentionally divulge information concerning a patient to anyone not directly involved in the patient's care.

4.2. discuss his/her patients in a public place and will take other precautions to ensure that she/he does not inadvertently pass on information regarding a patient.

As a medical student you will have access to information about patients, which they will expect to be kept confidential. Some of this you will obtain directly from patients or their relatives when you take histories. Other information will be available to you because you are given access to the patient's medical records as part of your training. This information should not be deliberately divulged to anyone not directly involved in the patient's care. You should also take care not to inadvertently pass on information about a patient. Think about who else may see your report or hear your conversations. You should not discuss your patients in a public place.

5. Students must not allow their personal beliefs to prejudice their patients' care.

Students will care for patients irrespective of their views about patients' lifestyles, culture, religion and beliefs, race, colour, gender, sexuality, disability, age, nationality, or social or economic status.

You are entitled to hold any beliefs that you wish but you must not allow these to interfere with your care of patients. This corresponds to the requirements in paragraph 5 of *Good Medical Practice*, GMC.

6. Students will act quickly to protect patients from risk if they have good reason to believe that they or a colleague may not be fit to practise.

6.1. The student will immediately report any concerns to a senior member of staff using the procedures for whistle blowing which are in force in the medical school.

You may see a health professional or a fellow student behaving in a way that is likely to lead to harm to patients. You should discuss this immediately with a senior person such as a tutor whom you trust. It is uncomfortable to be a whistleblower but it is important and your professional duty not to ignore behaviour if you know it to be dangerous or reckless. Where necessary you should contact a professional organisation, or the GMC for advice.

6.2. Medical students should strive for high standards in their professional lives and their conduct should reflect this.

7. The student will take all of the opportunities provided to develop his/her professional knowledge and skills.

The student will be expected to:

7.1. attend all of the compulsory teaching sessions.

7.2. inform the medical school as soon as possible of the reason if s/he is unable to attend a compulsory session.

7.3. complete and submit course work and assignments on time.

7.4. be conscientious in his/her approach to self-directed learning.

7.5. endeavour to contribute effectively to any learning group of which he/she is a part.

7.6. respond positively to reasonable feedback on his/her performance and achievements.

7.7. immediately inform the medical school of factors that might affect his/her performance so that appropriate action can be taken.

7.8. carry out examinations (including intimate examinations where necessary and when a chaperone is present) on patients of both sexes.

This corresponds to the requirement in *Good Medical Practice* – Keep your professional knowledge and skills up to date.

At this stage you are acquiring knowledge and skills rather than maintaining them but the principle is the same. Learning is a professional duty. Reading up on the patients you have seen and practising your clinical skills is an essential part of your life as long as you remain within the medical profession. Failure to attend compulsory teaching sessions is a breach of professional standards.

8. The student will recognise the limits of his/her professional competence.

8.1. The student will not hesitate to ask for help and advice when needed.

This may appear obvious to you but there is a temptation to undertake tasks or give advice beyond your level of competence. If in doubt ask for help.

9. The student will be honest and trustworthy in all matters.

9.1. All forms of academic cheating and plagiarism are unacceptable and may result in disciplinary proceedings.

This corresponds to the requirement in *Good Medical Practice* – Be honest and trustworthy.

This applies to your clinical encounters and has wider implications. If you are not trustworthy in your academic life it will be difficult to be trustworthy in the clinical setting.

10. The student will work with colleagues in the ways that best serve patients' interests.

Students will:

10.1. acknowledge that health care is dependent on effective co-operation between all members of the team.

10.2. attempt to ensure that they maintain good relationships with the other health professionals caring for the patient.

10.3. treat other healthcare professionals, staff and other members of the university and fellow students with respect.

Health care is dependent on effective co-operation between all members of the team. Even as a student you must ensure that you maintain good relationships with the other health professionals caring for the patient.

11. The student undertakes to provide feedback on the usefulness, significance and effectiveness of all aspects of the course, including teaching.

11.1. The student will complete such evaluation tools as are agreed between the medical school and the student body.

The medical school makes every effort to ensure that the course you are undertaking is of the highest quality by a process of continuous quality enhancement. If this is to be effective, the medical school needs timely and honest feedback on the course highlighting what worked well and what needs to be changed. Your opinion is important.

12. The student will permit the processing of information about any Fitness to Practise procedure in which s/he is involved.

The GMC and CHMS are currently looking at how best to improve student fitness to practise and are in the process of consultation on FtP issues. The Charter will be reviewed and updated following the consultation, if necessary.

Appendix 2: The core outcomes of basic medical education

The principles of professional practice

The principles of professional practice set out in *Good Medical Practice* must form the basis of medical education:

- *Good clinical care*: Doctors must practise good standards of clinical care, practise within the limits of their competence, and make sure that patients are not put at unnecessary risk.
- *Maintaining good medical practice*: Doctors must keep up to date with developments in their field and maintain their skills.

- *Relationships with patients*: Doctors must develop and maintain successful relationship with their patients.
- *Working with colleagues*: Doctors must work effectively with their colleagues.
- *Teaching and training*: If doctors have teaching responsibilities, they must develop the skills, attitudes, and practices of a competent teacher.
- *Probity*: Doctors must be honest.
- *Health*: Doctors must not allow their own health or condition to put patients at risk.

The following curricular outcomes are based on these principles. They set out what is expected of graduates. All curricula must include curricular outcomes that are consistent with those set out below.

Outcomes

Graduates must be able to do the following.

Good clinical care

(a) Know about and understand the following:
 (i) Our guidance on the principles of good medical practice and the standards of competence, care, and conduct expected of doctors in the UK.
 (ii) The environment in which medicine is practised in the UK.
 (iii) How errors can happen in practice and the principles of managing risks.
(b) Know about, understand, and be able to apply and integrate the clinical, basic, behavioural, and social sciences on which medical practice is based.
(c) Be able to perform clinical and practical skills safely.
(d) Demonstrate the following attitudes and behaviour:
 (i) Recognise personal and professional limits, and be willing to ask for help when necessary.
 (ii) Recognise the duty to protect patients by taking action if a colleague's health, performance, or conduct is putting patients at risk.

Maintaining good medical practice

(a) Be able to gain, assess, apply, and integrate new knowledge and have the ability to adapt to changing circumstances throughout their professional life.

(b) Be willing to take part in continuing professional development to make sure that they maintain high levels of clinical competence and knowledge.

(c) Understand the principles of audit and the importance of using the results of audit to improve practice.

(d) Be willing to respond constructively to the outcomes of appraisal, performance review, and assessment.

Relationships with patients

(a) Know about and understand the rights of patients.

(b) Be able to communicate effectively with individuals and groups.

(c) Demonstrate the following attitudes and behaviour:

   (i) Accept the moral and ethical responsibilities involved in providing care to individual patients and communities.

  (ii) Respect patients regardless of their lifestyle, culture, beliefs, race, colour, gender, sexuality, disability, age, or social or economic status.

 (iii) Respect the right of patients to be fully involved in decisions about their care, including the right to refuse treatment or to refuse to take part in teaching or research.

 (iv) Recognise their obligation to understand and deal with patients' health care needs by consulting them and, where appropriate, their relatives or carers.

Working with colleagues

(a) Know about, understand and respect the roles and expertise of other health- and social-care professionals.

(b) Be able to demonstrate effective team-working and leadership skills.

(c) Be willing to lead when faced with uncertainty and change.

Teaching and training

(a) Be able to demonstrate appropriate teaching skills.

(b) Be willing to teach colleagues and to develop their own teaching skills.

Probity

Graduates must demonstrate honesty in all areas of their professional work.

Health

Graduates must be aware of the importance of their own health, and its effect on their ability to practise as a doctor.

(From *Tomorrow's Doctors*, 2nd edition, General Medical Council (GMC), 2002.)

Appendix 3: Good medical practice

The duties of a doctor

Patients must be able to trust doctors with their lives and health. To justify that trust, you must show respect for human life and you must:

- Make the care of your patient your first concern.
- Protect and promote the health of patients and the public
- Provide a good standard of practice and care
  - Keep your professional knowledge and skills up to date
  - Recognise and work within the limits of your competence
  - Work with colleagues in the ways that best serve patients' interests
- Treat patients as individuals and respect their dignity
  - Treat patients politely and considerately
  - Respect patients' right to confidentiality
- Work in partnership with patients
  - Listen to patients and respond to their concerns and preferences
  - Give patients the information they want or need in a way they can understand
  - Respect patients' right to reach decisions with you about their treatment and care
  - Support patients in caring for themselves to improve and maintain their health
- Be honest and open and act with integrity
  - Act without delay if you have good reason to believe that you or a colleague may be putting patients at risk
  - Never discriminate unfairly against patients of colleagues
  - Never abuse your patients' trust in you or the public's trust in the profession.

How good medical practice applies to you

It is your responsibility to be familiar with Good Medical Practice and to follow the guidance it contains. It is guidance, not a statutory code, so you must use your judgement to apply the principles to various situations you will face as a doctor, whether or not you routinely see patients. You must be prepared to explain and justify your decisions and actions. In Good Medical Practice the terms "you must" and "you should" are used in the following ways:

- "You must" is used for an overriding duty or principle.
- "You should" is used when we are providing an explanation of how you will meet the overriding duty.
- "You should" is also used where the duty or principle will not apply in all situations or circumstances, or where there are factors outside your control that affect whether or how you can comply with the guidance.

(From *Good Medical Practice – Guidance from the GMC*, 2006).

Appendix 4: Work experience contacts

National Association of Volunteer Bureaux
New Oxford House
16 Waterloo Street
Birmingham
B2 5UG
Tel: 0121 633 4555

The National Centre for Volunteering
Regent's Wharf
8 All Saints Street
London N1 9RL
Tel: 020 7713 6161

Community Service Volunteers
237 Pentonville Road
London
N1 9NJ
Tel: 020 7278 6601

Appendix 5: Website addresses for UK medical schools

These sites give up-to-date information on contacts, admissions, entry requirements, and the course structure.

Aberdeen http://www.abdn.ac.uk/medicine
Barts & the London Queen Mary's http://www.smd.qmul.ac.uk
Birmingham http://medweb.bham.ac.uk
Brighton and Sussex http://www.bsms.ac.uk
Bristol http://www.bristol.ac.uk/fmd
Cambridge http://www.medschl.cam.ac.uk/
Cardiff http://www.cardiff.ac.uk/medicine
Dundee http://www.dundee.ac.uk/medicalschool
East Anglia http://www.med.uea.ac.uk
Edinburgh http://www.mvm.ed.ac.uk
Glasgow http://www.gla.ac.uk/faculties/medicine
Guy's, King's & St Thomas's, London http://www.kcl.ac.uk/schools/medicine
Hull-York http://www.hyms.ac.uk
Imperial College, London http://wwwfom.sk.med.ic.ac.uk/medicine
Keele http://www.keele.ac.uk/depts/ms
Leeds http://www.leeds.ac.uk/medicine
Leicester http://www.le.ac.uk/sm/le
Liverpool http://www.liv.ac.uk/medicine
Manchester http://www.medicine.manchester.ac.uk
Newcastle http://medical.faculty.ncl.ac.uk
Nottingham http://www.nottingham.ac.uk/medical-school
Oxford http://www.medsci.ox.ac.uk
Peninsula http://www.pms.ac.uk/pms
Queen's University, Belfast http://www.qub.ac.uk/cm
Sheffield http://www.shef.ac.uk/medicine
Southampton http://www.som.soton.ac.uk
St Andrew's http://medicine.st-and.ac.uk
St George's, London http://www.sgul.ac.uk
Swansea http://www.gemedicine.swan.ac.uk
University College, London http://www.ucl.ac.uk/medicalschool/index. shtml
Warwick http://www2.warwick.ac.uk/fac/med

Appendix 6: Access to medicine courses

The course at King's Lynn is the most widely accepted, although many other places run good courses. Be careful though: not all "access to medicine/ science" courses are deemed as meeting academic entry requirements by different medical schools. Some courses are not accepted by any medical schools.

College of West Anglia, King's Lynn:
http://www.col-westanglia.ac.uk/

City College, Norwich:
http://www.ccn.ac.uk/ccn3/general/co....asp?extra=125

Sussex Downs:
http://www.sussexdowns.ac.uk/xpurpos...o-medicine.asp

Manchester College of Arts and Technology:
http://www.mancat.ac.uk/adult/course...le&leaflet=103

Lambeth College:
http://www.lambethcollege.ac.uk/cour...cfm?cit_id=492

City College Islington:
http://www.candi.ac.uk/

Soton WAMP course:
http://www.som.soton.ac.uk/prospectu...mp/default.asp

St Georges Foundation to Medicine:
http://www.sgul.ac.uk/students/under...r-medicine.cfm

University of Sheffield Foundation year to Medicine:
http://www.shef.ac.uk/prospectus/cou...mp;kw=medicine

University of Nottingham Foundation year to Medicine:
http://www.lincoln.ac.uk/home/course...ence/index.asp

Bradford Clinical Sciences:
http://www.brad.ac.uk/acad/clinsci

Access course for entry to Liverpool:
http://doris.ucsm.ac.uk/access/access1.htm

Access course for entry to King's College London
http://www.kcl.ac.uk

Appendix 7: Useful general medical websites

Academy of Medical Royal Colleges: www.aomrc.org.uk

British Medical Association: www.bma.org.uk

Department of Health: www.doh.gov.uk

General Medical Council: www.gmc-uk.org

Medical Research Council: www.mrc.ac.uk

Medlink Conferences: www.medlink-uk.com

National Institute of Clinical Excellence: www.nice.org.uk

Royal Society: www.royalsoc.ac.uk

Royal Society of Medicine: www.roysocmed.ac.uk

Index

Lightning Source UK Ltd.
Milton Keynes UK
UKOW06f2125201214

243469UK00006B/136/P